BOA

Risk: what's your perspective?

A guide for healthcare professionals

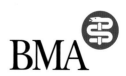

Editorial board

British Library Cataloguing-in-Publication Data.
A catalogue record for this book is available from the British Library.
ISBN-10: 1-905545-58-4
ISBN-13: 978-1-905545-58-2

Cover photograph: Getty Images Creative.

Board of Science

This report was prepared under the auspices of the Board of Science of the British Medical Association, whose membership for 2011/12 was as follows:

Professor David Haslam	President
Dr Steve Hajioff	Chairman of the Representative Body
Dr Hamish Meldrum	Chairman of Council
Dr Andrew Dearden	Treasurer
Mr Tony Bourne	Chief Executive
Dr Kate Bullen	Deputy Chairman of Council
Professor Averil Mansfield	Chairman, Board of Science
Mr Ram Moorthy	Deputy Chairman, Board of Science
Dr Peter Dangerfield	
Dr Shreelata Datta	
Dr Lucy-Jane Davis	
Dr Louise Harding	
Professor David Katz	
Dr Peter Maguire	
Professor Michael Rees	
Dr Philip Steadman	
Dr David Wrigley	
Dr Richard Jarvis	Public Health Medicine Committee
Dr Andrew Thomson	Deputy Member

Approval for publication was recommended by the BMA Board of Professional Activities on 1 December 2011.

Acknowledgements

The Association is grateful for the help provided by the BMA committees and outside experts and organisations. We would particularly like to thank:

Dr Julie Barnett (Reader in Healthcare Research, Brunel University)

Professor Baruch Fischhoff (Howard Heinz University Professor, Department of Social and Decision Sciences and Department of Engineering and Public Policy, Carnegie Mellon University)

Professor Nick Pidgeon (Professor of Environmental Psychology and Director of the Understanding Risk Research Group, Cardiff University)

Professor David Spiegelhalter (Winton Professor of the Public Understanding of Risk, Centre for Mathematical Sciences, University of Cambridge).

Declaration of interest
There were no competing interests with anyone involved in the research and writing of this report. For further information about the editorial secretariat or Board members please contact the BMA Science and Education department which holds a record of all declarations of interest: info.science@bma.org.uk

---

FOREWORD

Managing health risks is integral to medical practice. Doctors will be familiar with the risks, benefits, and uncertainties surrounding the common procedures and treatments of their chosen specialty, and an important aspect of the patient-doctor encounter is the communication of risk. As important as understanding the statistics behind various health risks is recognising the social and psychological factors that influence our perception of risk.

Health risks can range from major public health events such as pandemic influenza, natural disasters and terrorist attacks, to lifestyle risks such as obesity, alcohol and tobacco use. There are also a range of risks encountered in the healthcare setting such as the risks of screening for cancer, adverse drug reactions, and acquiring healthcare associated infections. Many of these health risks and their management have been of interest to the BMA and its Board of Science, which has produced a number of publications on these topics.

The BMA published *Living with risk* in 1987 and was awarded the 1988 Science Book Prize by the Science Museum. In the intervening decades, a number of significant public health events have helped to reshape how we respond to and perceive risks, and a wealth of new research has offered a greater depth of knowledge concerning risk management and communication. At its 2010 Annual Representative Meeting (ARM), the BMA resolved to update *Living with risk* to reflect our understanding of risk in the 21st century.

Risk: what's your perspective aims to help doctors understand risk and provide an overview of the major health risks faced by the UK population. It aims to help doctors communicate risk to their patients and the public, reviewing effective risk communication strategies, and outlining common attitudes and perceptions of risk.

Averil O. Mansfield

Professor Averil Mansfield
Chairman, BMA Board of Science

Risk: what's your perspective? A guide for healthcare professionals

CONTENTS

INTRODUCTION

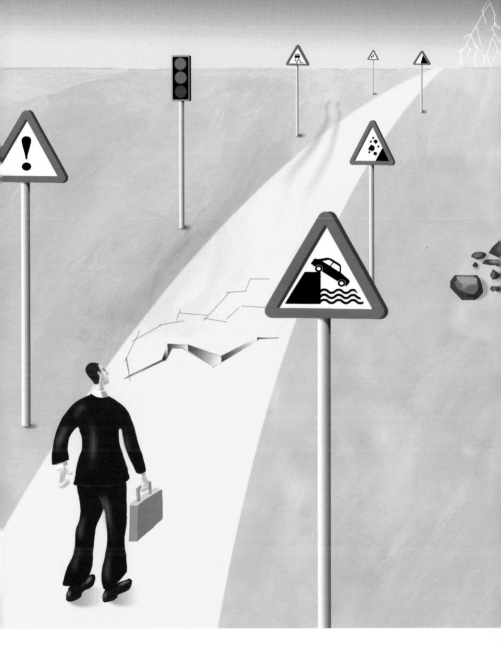

1.   INTRODUCTION

Doctors are faced with risk in their daily practice, perhaps more than any other profession: from immediate and serious threats to life, to weighing the risks of one treatment against another, to helping patients manage their exposure to the risks in their own lives. In an increasingly risk aware but risk averse culture,[1-2] doctors are well-placed to inform their patients, and help them to understand health risks. They have far greater experience of evaluating some common and rare risks than most, which gives them a unique and valuable perspective on this topic.

Patients often ask doctors: "is it safe?" – to which the answer is never straightforward or uncomplicated. The reality that nothing carries definitively zero risk, or is absolutely "safe", can be difficult to communicate. In the clinical setting, understanding risk, being fluent in the language of risk, and communicating in a meaningful way to patients, are essential skills for every doctor.

It is unsurprising that expert risk assessments rarely reflect public perceptions of these same risks. A common perception is that there are more risks today than in the past, and that most of these risks are unacceptably high.[1-2] In some instances individuals are willing to tolerate extremely high levels of risk, for example when mountain climbing, riding a motorcycle, or smoking cigarettes. In other cases there is seemingly no threshold of acceptable risk, for example when regulating exposure to nuclear radiation. The changing landscape of legal liability for the health of consumers, employees and citizens as well as the prospect of litigation and compensation claims, is compelling employers, companies, institutions and governments to adopt ever more stringent health and safety regulations.

That is not to say that these exaggerated or dismissive perceptions of the risks are unfounded or irrational. Public reactions to risk – which at first sight seem disproportionate compared to expert assessments and the quantitative information available – are underpinned by the cultural, social and psychological dimensions of risk perception. These rightly inform the choices individuals make about acceptable health risks in their lives.

As risks become increasingly complex and abstract, quantitative, empirical information is becoming essential and integral to the understanding and management of risk. In short, statistical and scientific literacy are indispensable tools for getting (and keeping) risk in perspective.

The original BMA publication *Living with risk*,[3] published in 1987, was awarded the 1988 Science Book Prize by the Science Museum. A limited edition was published in 1990. In the intervening two decades, much has changed in terms of our understanding and perceptions of risk – including risk communication, management, measurement, and prevention. New risk factors have emerged, new lessons have been learned from health risks, and a greater understanding of commonly recognised risk factors has been gained. At the 2010 Annual Representative Meeting (ARM), BMA members unanimously passed a resolution to update the Association's work in this area.

An overview of the report

This report seeks to provide an introduction to understanding risk in medicine and public health in a way that is relevant to doctors in their everyday practice, whether in the context of the patient-doctor relationship, or public health communications. Understanding the expert and technical assessment of risk, as well as recognising risk perceptions and how patients and the public respond to risk, will improve risk communication with patients and the public.[1]

The first chapter examines people's attitudes to risk, and provides an overview of risk concepts – including understanding and measuring risk, risk and uncertainty, and risk communication. It also discusses the role of medical and health risk information in the wider context of risk perception and risk evaluation in society, drawing on case studies to illustrate these concepts.

The second chapter considers the different types and sources of health risks that people may face, starting with the most common sources of risk to health in everyday life, from tobacco and alcohol use to occupational and transport risks. It goes on to explore everyday medical risks as well as risks that arise in the healthcare environment, and concludes by outlining some of the environmental risks, man-made and natural, that impact on population health.

Doctors will be familiar with and already use the recommended and effective risk management strategies for a variety of health risks that they encounter in caring for patients (eg providing advice on safe sex, administering vaccinations, adhering to high standards of hygiene in the clinical setting). There will, however, be risks which doctors are less familiar with, such as those associated with chemical hazards, emerging technologies, and natural disasters. This report outlines some of the general principles of risk management, but does not provide a comprehensive account of every risk management option for every identified health risk within the report. Where relevant, signposting is provided for additional information.

This report primarily aims to help doctors understand health risks and put risk in perspective. It should not be taken as an encyclopaedic account of the major health risks of 21st century life. It endeavours to equip doctors with an understanding of the basic concepts of risk, to provide a sense of the most common – and commonly feared – health risks, and to introduce strategies and tools for successful risk communication with patients and the public. Suggested further reading is highlighted throughout the report and in the sources of further information section.

RISK: KEY CONCEPTS

2.   RISK: KEY CONCEPTS

Risk is inherently complex. Understanding health risks involves the intersection of many disciplines: from medicine, biomedical research and epidemiology, to psychology, decision science and the social sciences. Attitudes to risk are influenced by perceptions and assumptions, and are not always compatible with medical evidence and statistical data. Understanding attitudes and perceptions, alongside how risk is quantified and assessed, are equally important and can aid risk communication and evaluation. Evidenced-based risk information has an important role to play in supporting this. Not only can a better scientific understanding of health risks influence perceptions of risk, evidenced-based risk information is also essential in identifying effective risk management strategies.

This chapter introduces a general definition of risk, and outlines the basic theories and concepts surrounding risk perception, measurement, communication, and evaluation. It includes:

- a lexicon for discussing risk
- common approaches to measuring risk
- appreciating uncertainty in risk
- common risk perception biases
- the social amplification of risk
- effective risk communication strategies
- risk evaluation processes
- the precautionary principle
- the dual use dilemma.

2.1.   Understanding risk

2.1.1.   Defining risk

Risk can have several meanings: its colloquial use implies danger and threat; in academic and economic contexts it is used to describe statistical concepts. Whereas benefit and harm describe tangible effects, in its basic form risk simply expresses the probability that an adverse event will occur, analogous to the likelihood, the odds or chance.[3] Risk, therefore, is inherently not a definite entity. People's attitudes to risk do not necessarily reflect this purely statistical definition, and are often at odds with how experts – including doctors and scientists – think about risk.

Why will one smoker eventually die from smoking-related illness, while another may not? This question summarises the probabilistic nature of risk. Information about a patient's lifestyle, environmental and genetic risk factors may re-categorise them into a high-risk group, or modify their absolute risk of premature death from a smoking-related cause from 50 to 99 per cent. While most would consider death virtually certain in this instance, the probability remains that for every 99 people who will die, one individual will survive. For the patient, it is never possible to know with certainty whether they will die from the disease, whatever their level of risk. They either will or they will not.

A risk lexicon can help to clarify these concepts:

Benefit: a positive outcome (eg improved health)

Harm: an adverse outcome (eg injury, illness, death)

Hazard: a circumstance or thing with the potential to cause harm (eg a boiling kettle, an industrial waste site)

Risk: the likelihood of harm

Risk factor: an agent or exposure that increases the risk of harm

Protective factor: an agent or exposure that decreases the risk of harm.[4]

To illustrate, the H1N1 virus is a hazard with the potential to cause harms, such as influenza symptoms and death in the population. The likelihood of being infected with the virus, or suffering from its effects, are the risk of infection and the risk of illness from H1N1 virus respectively. Risk factors that increase the risk of infection or illness include young age and poor hand hygiene. A protective factor that reduces the risk of infection or illness includes vaccination against the virus.

Defining risk can be complex, as is the case with smoking and ill health. While smoking increases the risk of illness and premature death, it also increases the risk of addiction, in this instance to nicotine. Addiction negatively impacts on the ability to quit smoking, reinforces the smoking habit, and so in itself increases the risk of disease and death.

Harm can be defined and quantified, and can be expressed in terms of death (mortality), illness or injury (morbidity). Harm can also be represented in more complex terms such as quality-adjusted life years (QALY) and disability-adjusted life years (DALY) lost.[a] These representations of harm reflect the quality of life and disease burden from health risks – the magnitude of the outcome – whereas risk only expresses the probability. An individual may have an equal risk of being injured at work as dying from stroke, but the magnitude of harm – injury or death – is considerably different. In quantifying harm, it is also possible to estimate its economic impacts, and assign a monetary cost to health risks.

2.1.2.   Measuring risk

Is it possible to know the level of risk for any given hazard? This question requires scientific investigation and statistical calculation, for which there are several approaches. Classical risk assessment refers to the technical and rational study of risk, and involves identifying, characterising and quantifying risk.[1] Doctors will be familiar with many of these research methods:

> **Scientific experimentation** in laboratories is one approach to measuring the likelihood of harm from a hazard. Laboratory experiments can be useful preliminary tests to measure the toxicity of new chemicals, for example, when it would be dangerous or unethical to perform these tests on humans. In a laboratory setting, individual variables can be manipulated in a controlled way to elucidate cause and effect, dose-response, probability of harm, mechanisms of action, and so on. Typically animals, such as rats and mice, are used in these experiments, which rely on the assumption of similar physiological responses occurring in humans.[3] The use of **computer modelling** to predict a range of possible outcomes is increasingly common in risk research. It is never easy to extrapolate from these controlled experiments to what might unfold when applied to humans.

---

a   DALY and QALY are two methods of quantifying harm to health
- DALY measures the gap between ideal and perfect health (in terms of life expectancy and healthy life years) and the actual health status of a current situation. It is the sum of years of life lost due to premature mortality (YLL) and years lived with disability (YLD): DALY = YLL + YLD.
- QALYs are a measure of life expectancy that take into account the quality of life of each year lived. QALY quantifies one year of life expectancy according to a scale of perfect health (1) and death (0), so that a year lived in ill-health will fall between 0 and 1, depending on the severity of illness or disability.

The **randomised controlled trial** (RCT) is the 'gold standard' study design in medical research. The primary outcome of a RCT is information about the benefits of an intervention or pharmaceutical treatment. These trials can also provide information relating to health risks as part of the study design. In the most robust form of the trial – the double-blind RCT – subjects are randomly assigned to the control (sometimes a placebo) or treatment group at the start of the study. The subjects and the researchers involved in the trial are unaware – blind – to the treatment the subjects are receiving. This system eliminates bias and other confounding factors. These trials are best at determining the effectiveness of new pharmaceuticals or medical treatments; but they are often only of limited value in public health research, where variables cannot be so easily controlled and manipulated.

Researchers can observe and record naturally-occurring events in a representative sample of the population using a **cohort study**. These studies follow a group of individuals over a period of time and record their data against a set of defined outcomes. An example of a cohort study is the Whitehall Study, which has followed 18,000 men in the British Civil Service since 1967. The original Whitehall study was followed by the Whitehall II Study, which was set up in 1985 to follow a further 10,000 men and women in the Civil Service, and led by Sir Michael Marmot at University College London. For these cohort studies, researchers have recorded information on diet, weight, smoking status, blood pressure and cholesterol, mental functioning, and many employment and socioeconomic factors to investigate the link between socioeconomic inequalities and health in participants. The major findings of this research have concluded that:

- a social gradient of health exists in industrialised societies, where the lowest socioeconomic class experiences the poorest health and the highest experiences the best
- experiencing stress in the workplace increases the risk of ill health in employees

- working in an environment of supportive managers and colleagues reduces sickness absence and improves health in general
- a high effort-to-reward imbalance increases the risk of coronary heart disease (CHD)
- secure jobs enhance health and wellbeing, whereas poorly-managed organisational changes harm health.

Case-control studies take a snapshot of two or more groups of individuals at a single point in time and compare them against each other. An example of a case-control study is the pioneering study of Richard Doll and Austin Bradford Hill in 1950, that compared the incidence of lung cancer in a group of smokers and non-smokers in London (see **Box 1**).[5] Case-control studies generally compare the histories of people with and without an outcome of interest, and as such they only provide information on relative and not absolute risks.

What cohort and case-control studies have in common is that they study large samples of the population, in order to determine levels of risk, rather than exclusively focusing on the casualties of a particular event, or patients with a particular disease.[6]

Exhaustive enumeration of, for example, deaths from particular diseases can be carried out using official national statistics. This provides a *rate* at which adverse events have occurred, for example in terms of number per 100,000 people per year, which in turn is used as an estimate of the underlying risk to which they were exposed.

Box 1 – determining the health risks of smoking
Richard Doll and Austin Bradford Hill first established the relationship between smoking and health in 1950, by comparing two groups of male patients in London hospitals: smokers and non-smokers. They found that smokers were significantly more likely to be diagnosed with lung cancer than non-smokers.[5]

To examine the relationship between smoking and lung cancer in greater detail, they went on to design a cohort study, and followed a group of doctors (made up of smokers, non-smokers and ex-smokers) throughout their lives and recording their general health profile, age at, and cause of death. This was one of the first studies to establish that smoking causes lung cancer. Fifty years later the cohort study continues and has provided a wealth of data on the relationship between smoking and health.

Professor Doll and his colleagues demonstrated that the risks of smoking extend far beyond lung cancer, and are associated with a range of cancers, cardiovascular and respiratory diseases. They found that half of all regular lifetime smokers would die prematurely due to their smoking habit, in a dose-dependent relationship according to the number of cigarettes smoked per day.

Over the course of the study, the research team witnessed a divergence in life expectancy between smokers and non-smokers. Lifelong smokers died ten years younger on average than lifelong non-smokers (**see Figure 1**). The research team found that quitting, after any length of time smoking, dramatically benefitted an individual's health. The earlier in life an individual quit smoking, the greater life expectancy they could anticipate.[7]

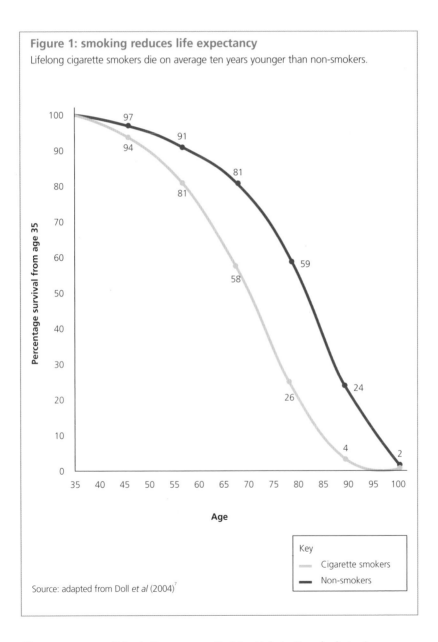

Figure 1: smoking reduces life expectancy

Lifelong cigarette smokers die on average ten years younger than non-smokers.

Source: adapted from Doll et al (2004)[7]

Some risks are so rare that they remain difficult to detect, even in a RCT or cohort study – especially when studying relatively common diseases in the first place.[8] The relatively small increase in the risk of cancer from exposure to radon radiation may be difficult to detect, for example, because the risk is small and because cancer is a common disease. Identifying a few extra cases of cancer with this specific cause in a population requires a large scale study with sufficient statistical power to detect these effects. The paradox with rare risks is that the more people exposed to a hazard, the more likely it is that harm will be observed – albeit in a very small proportion of all individuals exposed. This is commonly seen in relation to post-marketing surveillance for the rare side effects of medicines (see **Box 2**).

Risks, risk factors and hazards are also difficult to identify. The further apart the effect is from the cause, the more difficult it is to establish an association between the two. It is simpler to study and conclude, for example, that falling while skiing increases the risk of a broken bone than it is to establish that a lifetime of excessive sugar consumption increases the risk of cardiovascular disease.

Box 2 – post-marketing surveillance of Avandia (rosiglitazone)
The importance of sufficiently powerful clinical trials and post-market surveillance to detect adverse reactions is highlighted in the case of the diabetes drug rosiglitazone.

Independent post-marketing data analysis after the drug had been licensed prompted concerns over a suspected link to an increased risk of myocardial infarction (heart attack).[9] Ten years after its initial approval by the Food and Drug Administration (FDA) and the European Medicines Agency (EMA), the drug has been withdrawn in Europe and is under investigation in the United States (US).[10-11]

Rosiglitazone was approved in Europe and the US with only limited data from clinical trials conducted over a short timescale, in accordance with existing regulatory protocols.[10] As is the case with every new drug, licensing decisions are based on clinical trial data that cannot fully predict the range of adverse reactions that may occur in a larger patient population. Post-marketing surveillance is essential for all drugs for this reason, especially those used for long-term conditions. Concerns were raised at the time regarding the ability to predict any long-term ill-health consequences of rosiglitazone use from the limited available clinical trial data. In response to these safety concerns, the EMA required that the drug's manufacturer, GlaxoSmithKline (GSK), undertake further post-marketing studies of the drug after its approval in 2000.[10-11]

In response, GSK commissioned the RECORD clinical trial to determine the safety of rosiglitazone, specifically with respect to cardiovascular outcomes. The trial design, however, did not have sufficient power to detect increases in risk of cardiovascular events compared to placebo or other available drugs to treat diabetes.[11] Through post-market surveillance, GSK observed an increase in cardiac events in patients prescribed the drug, which was reported to the FDA and EMA in 2006.[10]

An independent meta-analysis of available data on rosiglitazone adverse events in 2007 found that the drug was "associated with a significant increase in the risk of myocardial infarction" in patients.[9] Similar observations were made by the World Health Organization (WHO).[10]

A 2010 US Senate finance committee report investigated the licensing of rosiglitazone and raised concern over the lack of evidence of its safety.[12]

In response to this new information, the EMA recommended that rosiglitazone be suspended from the market in 2010, stating that the "benefits of rosiglitazone no longer outweigh its risks".[13] The UK Commission on Human Medicines similarly advised the Medicines and Healthcare products Regulatory Agency (MHRA) to withdraw the drug. The FDA decided to implement a risk evaluation and mitigation strategy (RIMS), restricting the use of rosiglitazone and requiring further tests to determine its safety.

2.1.3.   Uncertainty

While it is possible to estimate a risk using statistical analysis of data, there is a degree of uncertainty associated with this. Requiring 100 per cent certainty would disqualify most if not all of medical practice and biomedical science. There is an element of uncertainty in all analyses based on data,[14] and researchers may express this as a range (confidence interval), attach a level of confidence that the results are not due to chance (significance testing),[15] or give a qualitative assessment of possible systematic biases in the estimates.

Uncertainty in predicting the risk of a likely future outcome can arise through a lack of knowledge or information. This is known as epistemic uncertainty. It is not possible, for example, to predict a patient's individual risk of developing type 2 diabetes without gathering information about their lifestyle and family history. Accurately modelling the spread of a communicable disease is only possible with reliable information on the size of the population, the mechanism and frequency of transmission, the prevalence and incidence of the disease, the level of immunity, and other relevant information.

Epistemic uncertainty can be reduced or eliminated through investigation and research. The quality of a study design and resulting quality of data will determine its ability to draw conclusions about a particular risk with any certainty. A large, well-designed cohort study involving 50,000 participants will yield a more accurate and precise estimate of risk than a small pilot study of 50 or 100 participants, which will have limited statistical power to detect rare and long-term delayed consequences of exposure to a hazard.

Uncertainty can also arise because of unpredictable variation, which is characterised by a random element. This is commonly known as aleatory uncertainty, and can be easily illustrated by the outcomes of tossing dice and drawing cards from a shuffled pack. When tossing dice, although the probability of a six appearing is known (one in six), it is not possible to predict that a six will appear on any given throw of the die. This unpredictable variation can also occur as a result of human error, such as a patient taking the incorrect dosage of a prescription medicine. Unlike epistemic uncertainty, this form of unpredictable uncertainty cannot be reduced through further investigation.

In practice, both types of uncertainty affect the ability to predict a likely outcome. The degree of acceptable uncertainty depends on the level of risk involved and the magnitude of potential harm (see **Box 3**).

Box 3 – risk and uncertainty: BSE
Bovine spongiform encephalopathy (BSE) was identified in 1986 as a novel infectious neurological degenerative disease affecting cattle. It was observed to be similar in nature to scrapie, which affects sheep and is transmitted by prions – a type of small protein.

A working party chaired by Sir Thomas Southwood was set up to determine whether the disease posed a threat to human health. The Southwood report published in 1989 concluded that, like scrapie, BSE was "unlikely" to transmit to humans and posed a negligible risk to human health.[16] The report recommended surveillance to rule out transmission to humans. The Spongiform Encephalopathy Advisory Committee (SEAC) reached the same conclusion in 1994. Its chair, Dr David Tyrell, advised the

---

Chief Medical Officer that "any risk as a result of eating beef or beef products is minute".[4]

The disease remained a serious health risk for cattle, however, and the Southwood report made a number of recommendations to reduce transmission among cattle. These included banning ruminant-derived meat and bone meal from cattle feed – an intensive farming practice known to transmit prions from sheep to cattle. Due to the perceived low risk to human health, these recommendations were not followed strictly in the farming industry.[4]

The first cases of transmission to humans were recognised through the surveillance programmes as variant CJD (vCJD). Due to the long incubation period before symptoms appeared (more than 15 years), there was – and remains – a high degree of *uncertainty* in the number of subclinically infected people and the escalation trajectory of the disease in the UK population. Estimates of the cases of vCJD that could be expected varied from a few hundred to more than 100,000.[17]

Since the 1990s there have been 173 confirmed cases of vCJD that were caused by consumption of BSE-infected beef or blood transfusion from a BSE-infected donor. The number of new cases peaked in 2000 and has been in decline since, but *uncertainty* remains as to whether a second wave of cases will be observed. Recent estimates of the prevalence of individuals subclinically infected with vCJD range from 0 to 60.8 people per 100,000 population,[18] broadly in agreement with an earlier study that estimated 25 cases per 100,000 population.[19]

Once the first cases of vCJD developed and were linked to BSE, the perception of risk was greatly heightened among the public. The safety of British beef came into question, and in 1996 the European Union (EU) banned the export of beef from the UK, a ban which was not lifted until 2006. Within the UK, a programme of selective cattle slaughter was introduced in 1996 to prevent cattle most at risk from BSE from entering the human or animal food chain. In 1997, the sale of beef on the bone was banned in the UK to further reduce the risk of transmission of BSE to humans.

2.2.   Risk perception and attitudes to risk

The origin of the word 'risk' is probably derived from the Greek *rhiza*: the danger of sailing too near to cliffs. The image that *rhiza* evokes – of changeable winds and turbulent seas – shares many similarities to the understanding of the meaning of risk today.[3] 'Risky' still implies hazard, danger, uncontrollable and unpredictable events, reckless and daring behaviour.

Awareness of the nature of a risk is critical to effectively managing it. Expert judgements help to quantify and characterise risks, whereas public perceptions of risk additionally reflect the social, cultural and institutional contexts within which these risks exist.[1] Discrepancies between expert assessments and lay perceptions exist for risks with strong associated social or cultural values, and expert assessments are not always successful in influencing public perceptions.[20] Risk perception is also influenced by unconscious cognitive processes, intuition, emotion and feelings.

If the perceived risk diverges significantly from the quantifiable likelihood of harm, individuals might unknowingly expose themselves to higher levels of risk than anticipated, or give up potential benefits for fear of experiencing harm. With vaccination and immunisation, if the perceived risks of vaccination are exaggerated compared to the known risks, there is a potential to forgo the benefits associated with its use (eg population and individual immunity to a disease). If the perceived risks of poor diet and physical inactivity are underestimated compared to the real risk of cardiovascular disease and obesity, an individual is likely to experience a higher than anticipated level of illness in the future.

Many people consider safety to be the opposite of risk, particularly in relation to health issues. The complete elimination of harm occurring is usually neither practicable nor possible. Safety does not correspond to zero risk, but to an acceptably low level of risk. It is up to society to debate and determine where the threshold of acceptable risk lies, and how this will impact on risk management practices, legal liability and restrictions to personal freedoms (see section 2.4.2).

2.2.1. Fright factors and the psychometric paradigm

The types of risk and how they are presented play an important part in how individuals react to different scenarios which may or may not cause them harm. These intuitive judgements about the riskiness of a hazard are known as the **psychometric paradigm**,[1, 21] and a number of factors that influence risk perception have been characterised.

Two dimensions of risk have been identified that particularly influence risk perception. The first is the dread factor – when a risk is perceived to be uncontrollable, potentially catastrophic, involuntary, and inequitable. The second is the unknown factor – when a risk is considered new, unfamiliar, has delayed consequences, is not directly observable, and is poorly understood by science.[1, 4] Other "fright factors" that tend to intensify a sense of danger from risk include: risks to pregnant women and children, the perceived lethality of the risk, lack of trust in the source of risk, and connotations of blame.[4, 22]

The sense of dread associated with a natural disaster such as a tsunami – its catastrophic, uncontrollable and inescapable nature – may lead to the perception that it is a greater risk than flooding, which in fact causes more death and destruction globally on an annual basis. The unfamiliarity of modern technologies such as genetically-modified food or nanotechnology may sometimes make them seem more threatening than everyday risks such as pesticide residues in food, or exposure to common chemicals.

Just as individuals overestimate high consequence risks, they are prone to underestimate common and familiar risks.[23] Factors that dampen the perception of risk include complexity, risks restricted to marginalised groups, risks that are in conflict with ideology or values, and personal responsibility and control over risks (eg individuals will accept 1,000 times greater risk if it is voluntary,[1] such as lifestyle and leisure risks).[1, 4, 23] Doctors will also be aware that patient perceptions of risk develop from previous experience, attitudes, values, beliefs, personality, and socio-demographic factors.[21-22, 24]

2.2.2.   Common perception biases

The way individuals intuitively understand risk is often very different to the statistical and scientific processes used to calculate the actual probability of an adverse event occurring. The brain makes use of mental strategies to simplify complex cognitive tasks such as decision-making and risk judgements. While these intuitive and learned decision-making shortcuts – known as **heuristics** – are often valid, they can also introduce systematic biases in judgements of risk of harm from a range of threats, and distort risk perception.[1, 4, 25] Experts – including doctors and scientists – are equally susceptible to these cognitive biases, especially when making judgements about risks outside their immediate areas of expertise.[1, 26] The following common perception biases frequently influence perceptions of risk among individuals:

Availability bias: the tendency to believe something is more likely to occur or more frequently occurring when information about it is readily recalled. Recent or salient events are easily recalled, however, even if relatively uncommon. Although the risk of death from aviation or rail travel (per passenger mile, or per journey) is very low, the public perception of this risk is often heightened due to availability bias – the ability to readily recall a similar event, such as a rail disaster – in part due to the intense media coverage of these rare events.[25]

Confirmation bias: the tendency to look for confirming evidence to support a belief rather than looking for disconfirming evidence (which is often more persuasive and definite) to refute it. Evidence that supports a preconception tends to be favoured over ambiguous or contrary evidence. Although evidence of the harms of alcohol consumption is far more conclusive and robust than the evidence of its benefits (see section 3.2.2), the latter is more valued because it confirms the public perception that alcohol consumption is a low risk activity.

Overconfidence bias: the tendency to act on incomplete information, where individuals often have more confidence in their own judgements, and believe that they carry a greater degree of certainty, than is often deserved. A central feature of gambling is the strength of confidence an individual has in their own decision-making over other players. Even when playing the lottery, confidence in choosing the correct numbers and influencing the outcome can be disproportionately strong, considering the extremely low probability of winning, and its entirely random nature.[1, 27]

Optimism bias: the tendency for an individual to believe that the risk of an adverse event happening to them is lower than average.[28-29] Optimism bias can hinder efforts to reduce lifestyle risk factors. Smokers are commonly known to underestimate their personal risk of lung cancer relative to non-smokers, and even relative to other smokers, including their ability to overcome addiction and quit smoking.[30]

Hindsight bias: the tendency to perceive the outcome of past events as being more predictable and foreseeable than they in fact were. A terrorist attack might be perceived as an inevitable consequence of a combination of variables. But accurately predicting (and preventing) a terrorist attack, and distinguishing between real threats and false alarms, is a major challenge.[31-33]

Probability neglect: the tendency to focus on the adverse outcome related to very low probability events, rather than the statistical probability of the outcome occurring. Events such as natural disasters and terrorist attacks are subject to probability neglect in the population because they evoke strong emotions including fear, anxiety or outrage. The imagery and salience of the catastrophic consequence exaggerate risk perception. In these circumstances, the public demand excessive preventive action and protection against very low probability events, and are willing to pay large sums in order to avoid them, even if the magnitude of risk does not justify the level of action.[34-35]

2.2.3. Risk perception and emotion

Two distinct cognitive systems are involved in making risk judgements – the experiential and analytic systems. The analytic system involves conscious reasoning, using probability, logic and risk assessment to arrive at a judgement about a particular risk. The experiential system involves automatic and intuitive cognitive processes, and relies on feelings and emotion, images and narratives to guide decisions and actions.[36]

Whereas the analytic system is slow and deliberative, the experiential system is rapid, instinctive and often subconscious. It precedes and guides the slower analytic decision-making system,[37-39] and is necessary for making accurate and appropriate decisions. A lack of emotion and feeling therefore leads to worse decision-making.[22, 40]

The experiential system can influence risk perception through associating risk events with positive or negative emotions – a process known as the **affect heuristic**. Whereas risk and benefit are positively correlated in the real world (taking a larger risk generally has the potential for a greater payoff), risk and benefit are negatively correlated in the mind.[1, 21] Events or behaviours are viewed positively when the benefits are perceived to be high, and the associated risk is assumed to be low. The opposite view is often taken when the perceived benefits are unclear or perceived to be low – the risk is assumed to be high or higher than acceptable.[39] This inconsistency is due to the strength of emotion associated with a risk or hazard, where positive emotion is associated with benefit, and negative emotion associated with risk.[21, 36, 39, 41]

The considerable and immediate social benefits of mobile phone technology, for example, led to its widespread uptake despite the health risks (if any) not being fully understood. Even if the health risks were greater, it is likely that the technology would still be embraced because of its associated benefits. The risks of driving are similarly widely accepted – up to a point – because of the mobility and convenience it affords. Situations in which the potential benefit and the risk are high therefore pose a dilemma and require a more complex judgement.[39] In these situations individuals tend to focus on positive or negative emotions attached to outcomes: if the benefits are likely to be substantial – for example by participating in a clinical trial pioneering a life-prolonging therapy for a terminal illness – people are likely to be more willing to accept higher levels of actual risk.

While the experiential system is effective at making quick, intuitive decisions about simple risks, it is not necessarily optimal for dealing with the more complex and abstract risks – for example risks that are psychologically distant such as the future risk of lung cancer from smoking,[36] or the risks of climate change to health.[37] This can lead to flawed judgements. Individuals may readily accept risks when they have immediate benefits and distant harms – for example the instant pleasure of fatty foods or cigarette smoking compared to the long-term risk of cardiovascular disease and cancer – a process known as **discounting**. This is commonly seen with adolescent attitudes to risk (see **Box 4**). Moral and social values influence risk-taking as much as accurate risk information (see section 2.2.5).

Box 4 – adolescent attitudes to risk

Risk aversion is the reluctance to take risks, even when the potential benefits are comparatively high. The attitudes of young people and adolescents to sunbed use, for example, suggest that although the majority are aware of the risks of skin damage and skin cancer, knowledge of future health risks is not necessarily a deterrent. The primary reason for using sunbeds in these age groups is the desire to look better, and a perception of tanned skin as healthy and attractive.[42]

Understanding adolescent attitudes to risk is complex. By age 15, adolescents have the same reasoning skills as adults, including the susceptibility to optimism bias.[26] But adolescents are still undergoing emotional development, which may contribute to poor risk judgements and behaviour (along with other factors such as social pressure and personal experiences).[26] Personality traits in adolescents such as impulsiveness, sensation-seeking, and a willingness to violate conventional norms, increase the likelihood of risky behaviours.[43] Peer group pressure also influences risk-taking behaviour,[44] and adolescents are aware that they sometimes engage in risky behaviours because they lack the ability to decline.[45]

Risk behaviours tend to occur in clusters. Adolescents who use sunbeds are also more likely to smoke, drink alcohol, and have an unhealthy diet.[46] Use of drugs, alcohol and tobacco is also clustered among adolescents: those who smoke are more likely to also drink alcohol or use drugs. Although 99 per cent of 11- 15 year olds recognise that drug, alcohol and tobacco use is bad for health,[47] peer behaviour, social skills, parenting and behavioural disinhibition are factors that influence the likelihood of using drugs, alcohol and tobacco.[47]

Parents are strong communicators of social and cultural norms, and parenting can have a positive influence on adolescent attitudes to risk. Positive parent-adolescent relationships protects against the uptake of smoking,[48] the development of eating disorders, unsafe sex and teenage pregnancy.[49] Other important factors that may influence exposure to, and attitudes towards, risk include socioeconomic disadvantage, low educational attainment, and family structure.[49]

2.2.4.   Framing

The way in which risk information is framed can influence an individual's response and interpretation. **Framing** is the expression of logically equivalent information in different ways[4, 50] – is the glass half empty or half full? This can lead to predictable and systematic shifts in preference depending on how the problem is framed.[51] Positive or negative framing can change an individual's perspective on a problem, influence their perception of risk, and their subsequent decisions and behaviours. When individuals lack an initial opinion (for example relating to a new or unfamiliar risk), they are more susceptible to framing effects.[1]

A simple illustration of framing in risk communication is the use of different reference points when discussing the same risk: the likelihood of death versus the chance of survival from cancer. Both describe the same risk. Individuals are usually unaware of the alternative frames for a given problem, and how these might affect their choices.[51]

Choosing an appropriate reference point can influence whether an outcome is considered a gain or a loss.[21] Outcomes framed as a loss, emphasising risk, are more effective in promoting behaviour change in general.[52] Outcomes framed as a gain, emphasising benefits, are effective in achieving prevention behaviour (for example emphasising the safety of seatbelts rather than the risks of not wearing them).[21]

Framing can be used to stimulate discourse: framing the risks of climate change in terms of future costs, as in the 2005 Stern report. This focused debate on the costs and benefits of different choices for mitigation and adaptation to climate change, rather than revisiting the science of climate change.[37]

It is recommended that outcomes should be expressed using positive and negative frames by describing what will happen to everyone (see section 2.3.4 for an example comparing treatment options for cervical cancer).

2.2.5.   The social amplification of risk framework

A question of great interest to experts and risk communicators is: why do risks with minor health consequences sometimes elicit strong public concern? How can the public perception of a risk diverge so significantly from expert risk assessment?

As well as psychological processes, risk perception is shaped by social, cultural and institutional processes.[53] Social contexts, peer group and cultural values, and ideological belief systems all mediate the individual or public response to risk.[1, 53-54] An awareness of how risk information is communicated to and interpreted by the public will help doctors in their own discussions with patients about these risks.

Risk information can be intensified or attenuated through these social and cultural processes.[4] One way of describing how an individual or community interprets risk information is through the **social amplification of risk framework**.[4] In this framework, risk messages are transmitted and filtered through 'amplification stations' – social networks, institutions, the news media, scientists and experts – that modify the message by adding, deleting or filtering information, and amplifying or attenuating the message. The media in particular play a critical role in articulating risks and shaping public opinion.[53] Individuals receiving the message must interpret and decode its meaning, influenced by their own social and cultural values, and psychological processes described in the earlier sections.[4, 53] It is inherently difficult, therefore, to predict how risk information will be received once in the public domain.

This process of amplification or attenuation is not without consequence and can have a number of knock-on effects – social, economic, regulatory, legislative – and can diminish public confidence in institutions. In some cases, the social amplification of risk can result in increased risk to the public (see **Box 5**).[53]

Box 5 – measles, mumps and rubella (MMR) vaccine safety

Public misperceptions of risk, once formed, can be difficult to change, and can have real health consequences. An example of this is the public perception of the link between the MMR vaccine and autism in young children that developed in the late 1990s.

The theory originated from a small study by Dr Andrew Wakefield, published in the Lancet journal in 1998.[55] This study reported a close temporal association between MMR vaccination and the onset of autism in young children, and implied that vaccination was the cause of autism.

The study was publicised widely in the international media and led to public concern about the MMR vaccine. The conclusions of the study were overstated on many occasions, with claims being made about the strength of the link between the MMR vaccine and autism that were not supported by the results.[56] All the other authors (except Wakefield) published retractions of the paper and distanced themselves from it. In 2010, the Lancet journal formally retracted the publication. Dr Wakefield was found guilty of fraudulent and ethical misconduct in relation to the study in 2010, and struck off the General Medical Council (GMC) Medical Register in the UK.[57-58]

Despite clear evidence that refuted the link with autism,[4] the media reporting of the article's claims had a significant impact on the public perception of the safety of the MMR vaccine. Doctors and the medical profession struggled to communicate the low risk of the vaccine in a way that the public, and parents in particular, would respect and accept.[4-6, 56]

The public perception of an increased risk of autism from the MMR vaccine led to a decrease in its uptake rate, from more than 90 per cent to fewer than 80 per cent of infants in the UK. This fall in vaccination uptake was followed by an increase in cases of measles in England and Wales, from 2,438 notifications in 1999 to a peak of 5,088 notifications in 2008 (see **Figure 2**).

Through the social amplification of risk, parents' values and the desire to protect their children from harm by withholding vaccination paradoxically resulted in an increased risk to their own children and the wider population from measles.

Figure 2: measles notifications and immunisations, 1995-2008.
As immunisation rates drop below the herd immunity threshold, over time a growing number of individuals in the community are susceptible to measles, and cases of measles begin to increase. For example, MMR immunisation rates dropped steadily to a low in 2003, which was followed by a rise in measles notifications after a three year lag from 2006.

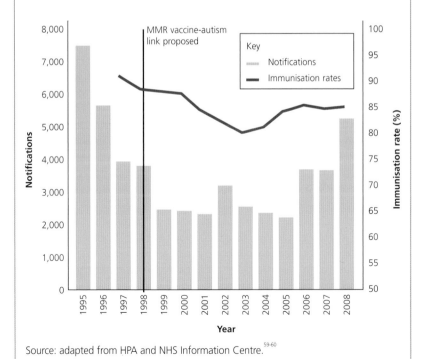

Source: adapted from HPA and NHS Information Centre.[59-60]

2.3.   *Communicating risk and uncertainty*

What is the best way to communicate about risks, hazards, outcomes and their uncertainties to patients and the public? The simple answer is that it depends, on the situation, on the audience, on the risk, and on the purpose of the communication. Is the goal, for example, to inform and increase understanding, achieve behaviour change, or avoid panic? Risk communication offers an opportunity to bridge the gap between expert assessments and lay perceptions of risk, and share understanding of an issue. The focus of this section is the discussion of communication methods that aid the understanding of health risks, avoid confusion, and put risk in perspective.

Doctors and medical experts are often the channel through which health risk information is relayed to the public. But doctors should be aware that they are only one source of health information. Patients and the public seek out information from many other channels, including television, the internet, news media, social networks, family and friends.[21] The majority of Americans, for example, now use the internet as their first source of health information, before their physician.[61]

Risk communication is a common feature of the patient-doctor consultation. Doctors often have two distinct and conflicting roles in risk communication: as the educator who provides independent, unbiased information to help patients and the public make informed choices and as the advocate who seeks to motivate positive behaviour change and improve the health of their patients and communities. These dual roles may necessitate different approaches to risk communication. The underlying goal should always be, however, to communicate risk information in a way that patients understand and accept as personally relevant, allowing them to make their own informed decisions.[20-21]

The medium and language of risk communication can be as important as the message itself.[4] Risk communication should aim to address knowledge, perceptions and behaviours. Patients and the public are interested in information relating to themselves and their illness.[62] They may only recall a small amount that is conveyed, and only in general terms.[63] Repetition and reinforcement of a message can aid awareness and recall.[64] Clarity in the message is key. Numerical, graphical, and verbal approaches can be adopted in risk communication.

The public want clear, definitive and unambiguous messages about the risk that they face.[54] Doctors and experts must balance this desire for clarity against the duty to provide accurate, relevant information, and reflecting the complexities and uncertainties surrounding some risks. Ultimately, accurate, unbiased and honest messages maintain the trust and credibility of doctors.

The best way for doctors to express risk is in a way that is meaningful, consistent and simple to understand. Key information to convey includes: an individual's absolute risk, an impression of the level of uncertainty, reference points for comparison, and graphical representations to increase clarity and perspective. Acknowledging some of the common risk perception biases and attitudes to risk can improve risk communication: empathetic language, narrative, and imagery can strengthen risk communication messages and motivate behaviour change.[21]

2.3.1. Approaches to communicating risk to patients and the public

Effective patient-doctor communications skills are essential for communicating risk to patients. The BMA publication *Communication skills education for doctors* (2004) highlights the importance of listening and interaction with patients, flexibility, and responsiveness in communication with patients. Consistency and clear take home messages can reinforce risk communication information. Emphasising two-way dialogue and a patient-centred approach to communication helps to build trust and improves patient decision-making.[20, 24] If doctors underestimate patient knowledge and perceptions of risk, the patient may disregard or consider the information provided by the doctor as irrelevant, and distance themselves from their health decisions.[20, 22]

The GMC considers good communication a cornerstone of the patient-doctor partnership, and describes effective communication as:

- listening to patients, asking for and respecting their views about their health, and responding to their concerns and preferences
- sharing with patients, in a way they can understand, the information they want or need to know about their condition, its likely progression, and the treatment options available to them, including associated risks and uncertainties

- responding to patients' questions and keeping them informed about the progress of their care
- making sure that patients are informed about how information is shared within teams and among those who will be providing their care.

Source: *Good Medical Practice* (GMC, 2006)

The shared decision-making model aims to achieve healthcare decisions based on mutual agreement. This model recommends that during the patient-doctor consultation, the health issue is defined and explained, options are presented and their risks, benefits and costs are discussed. Patient values are explored, and patient understanding is established. Finally, the doctor can offer recommendations and help the patient to reach a decision.[22]

Risk communication should aim to provide the necessary information and context in order for individuals to make informed choices. Individuals generate intuitive theories about risk based on the knowledge available to them, so that they feel competent in making decisions and participating in public debate – these are known as **mental models**.[22] Where mental models are incomplete or incorrect, doctors and risk communicators should aim to offer new ways of thinking about risks and their causes, so that individuals can integrate new information into a mental model in a way that is coherent and relevant to them. Doctors should aim to reinforce the correct elements of the theory, bridge gaps between lay and expert models, correct misconceptions, and identify the information and concepts most relevant to the patient.[21]

Public awareness and knowledge can vary from issue to issue, and communication strategies should be tailored to each. **Strategic listening** is a process that can be used to shape communications and more effectively address what the public need and want to know on a given risk.[21, 37, 65] Rather than approaching risk communication as a standard format, strategic listening helps communicators identify what information is important to a given issue, and tailor communication strategies accordingly. Strategic listening involves collaboration between natural, social and decision scientists. Surveys and in-depth interviews are used to identify knowledge gaps, what matters to different groups of people, and what information they feel is relevant or unclear. These findings can be incorporated into medical or scientific communications. After dissemination, the communications' impacts can be evaluated and used to improve future communication strategies. The research might find, for example in the case of climate change, that the public may feel that they have a general awareness of the issue, but are unsure of the different choices available to them to engage in mitigation or adaptation. In other cases, such as nanotechnology, they may lack basic knowledge about the technology and its risks.[37]

An example of strategic listening in the healthcare setting is the evaluation of the use of prescription drug fact boxes to improve patient understanding of the benefits and side effects of medication in the United States, where direct-to-consumer advertising of prescription drugs is common. Patients and consumers require efficacy and safety data about prescription drugs in order to make informed decisions. They are typically provided with a list of all possible side effects, and little data on drug efficacy.[66] The Dartmouth Veterans Administration Outcomes Group developed and evaluated a drug facts box designed to include the most relevant information about the benefits and side effects of a drug relative to control or placebo. Compared to standard drug information, patients and consumers were able to understand the data presented, found it useful, were less likely to overestimate a drug's benefits, and were better able to objectively compare two drugs.[66] The FDA Risk Communication Advisory Committee recommends the use of prescription fact boxes in communication and marketing to patients and consumers.[21, 66-67]

As new risks emerge it is necessary to establish professional expertise, legitimacy and authority over other interested parties. An example of this process would be during the 'tobacco wars', where the medical academic community and tobacco industry were in competition to establish authority and legitimacy over evidence of the effects of tobacco smoke on health. A current example is the challenge to scientific legitimacy surrounding climate change and its environmental and health risks (see section 3.5.6).

The 'Back to sleep' campaign is an example of successful public communication of medical research findings about infant sleeping position and risk of sudden infant death syndrome (SIDS) (see **Box 6**).

Box 6 – public communication and sudden infant death syndrome
While overall infant mortality is very low in the UK, SIDS is one of the leading causes of death in otherwise healthy infants. Until recently, the cause and risk factors for SIDS were largely unknown, and SIDS research was characterised by inconclusive and conflicting results.

Although a few studies suggested that the prone infant sleeping position increased the risk of SIDS, this was not widely recognised as a risk factor until the late 1980s and early 1990s. In the UK, the 1989 Avon study of SIDS identified sleeping position as a risk factor. The "Back to Sleep" public health campaign that followed aimed to communicate the risk of the prone sleeping position to parents, and recommended that infants be put to sleep on their backs. The campaign was very successful, and by 2004 annual deaths from SIDS had decreased by up to 70 per cent in some countries, and by over 50 per cent in the UK (see **Figure 3**).[6, 68-70] The main cause of SIDS deaths is now due to co-sleeping with parents and associated risk factors (alcohol, sleeping on sofas, and overcrowded housing).

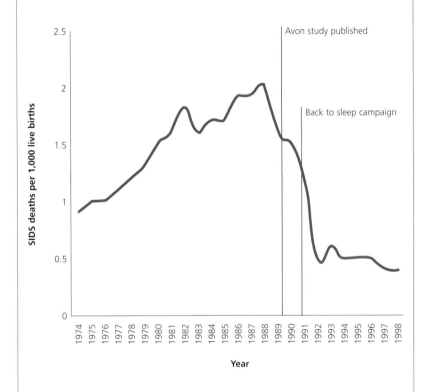

Figure 3: SIDS mortality in the UK, 1974-1998
SIDS decreased sharply following the 1991 'Back to Sleep' campaign in England and Wales.

Avon study published

Back to sleep campaign

SIDS deaths per 1,000 live births

Year

Source: Modified from Gilbert et al (2005).[70]

2.3.2.   Trust

Trust is essential for effective communication. Public trust in risk information depends heavily on the source – experts, government, industry, media – and is crucial to the public response to risks.[71] A number of factors are important in building public trust:

- proactive public engagement
- responsibility demonstrated through action
- transparency in decision-making, information sources and conflicts of interest
- acknowledgement of uncertainty and complexity.[4]

Of all professions and institutions, the medical profession enjoys the highest level of public trust, and academic science is also a highly trusted institution (least trusted are tabloid newspapers, members of parliament and government departments).[37, 54, 72] As trusted members of society, doctors and scientists are well-placed to communicate risk messages to the public, and have a responsibility to maintain public trust. This requires the continual demonstration of competence, independence, credibility, and a lack of self-interest or conflicts of interest.[3, 54]

Building trust in the context of the patient-doctor relationship requires developing an open, reciprocal relationship.[20] *Trust* typically develops from the personal experiences of the patient (eg in their interactions with individual healthcare professionals) whereas *confidence* typically relates to systems, institutions and governance (eg the healthcare system).[73] Patients can therefore simultaneously have trust in the doctors and nurses who care for them, but lack confidence in the healthcare system as a whole, or vice versa.

2.3.3.   Numerical information

The way in which risk is expressed in numerical terms can influence its understanding, and poor numeracy skills among the public can be a barrier to risk communication.

The following question was asked in a survey of the general adult population: *"Which of the following numbers represents the biggest risk of getting a disease: 1 in 100, 1 in 1000, 1 in 10?"* Twenty-five per cent of Americans and 28 per cent of Germans answered incorrectly.[74] Less numerate individuals rely more on the experiential system (ie emotion, narratives and mood states), involve the analytic system less in their risk perception and decisions, and are more sensitive to information about harms and adverse effects associated with risks.[21, 75]

Absolute risk refers to the actual probability of a person within the population experiencing a given harm – for example a 2 per cent chance, 1 in 50 chance, or 20 per 1,000 population, which are all equivalent.

Relative risk is used to compare two scenarios, for example the 50 per cent increase in risk of premature death in smokers, compared to non-smokers. Relative risk can be misleading because it lacks context – individuals (including doctors) tend to exaggerate or overestimate the magnitude of any effect.[62, 76] Relative risk is rarely useful in helping to understand risk, unless when comparing two clearly defined alternatives, as with the smoking example, and in conjunction with information on absolute risks.[50] It may be that the risk has doubled, but whether it doubles from an absolute risk of 1 in a million to 2 in a million, or from 1 in 3 to 2 in 3, is important information to know.

To illustrate the difference between absolute and relative risk, see **Figure 4**. A woman might discover that she is at twice the risk of multiple sclerosis and breast cancer than the average female population in the UK. For both conditions, her risk has doubled. The absolute risks of developing breast cancer or multiple sclerosis, are considerably different. Her risk of multiple sclerosis is increased from 1 in 188 to 2 in 188; whereas her risk of breast cancer is increased from 1 in 8 to 2 in 8.

Relative risk information alone, therefore, can be misleading. Mammography has been shown to reduce the relative risk of mortality from breast cancer by 20-25 per cent, which corresponds to a reduction from five to four women per 1,000, or a 0.1 per cent absolute risk reduction.[77-79] Although a 25 per cent reduction in relative risk appears impressive, because mortality from breast cancer in the general population is low (5 per 1,000 women), the absolute reduction is correspondingly small. A 2010 study found that when this relative risk was communicated to a representative sample of 5,000 European women, nearly all (92%) overestimated the benefit of mammography screening by up to 100-fold, or did not know.[77, 80] More than a quarter of British women interpreted the relative risk to mean that, for every 1,000 women, 200 fewer would die from breast cancer. Doctors can make the same mistake: nearly a third interpreted the relative risk to mean that 25 or 250 fewer women would die as a result of mammography screening.[77] See section 3.4.4 for further discussion of the complexities of assessing the risks and benefits associated with mammography screening.

Figure 4: absolute risk versus relative risk
The relative risk doubles for multiple sclerosis (left) and breast cancer (right), however, the increase in absolute risk is substantially different in the two examples.

Multiple sclerosis

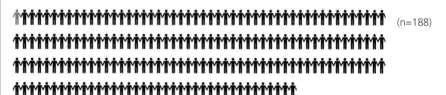

absolute risk: 1 in 188

risk doubles

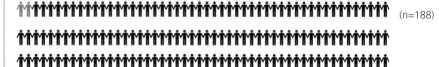

absolute risk: 2 in 188

Source: www.cancerresearchuk.org and www.mstrust.org.uk (accessed April 2011).

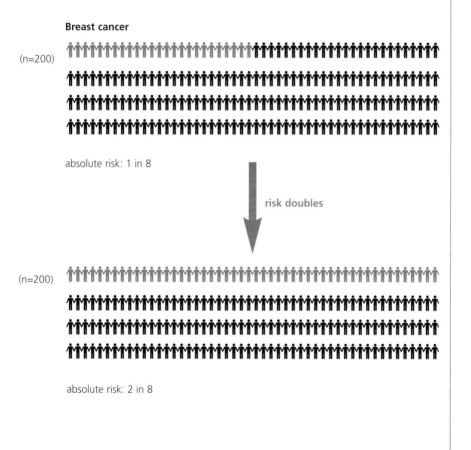

Breast cancer

(n=200)

absolute risk: 1 in 8

risk doubles

(n=200)

absolute risk: 2 in 8

What is the best method for translating risk probabilities calculated from population studies into information that is meaningful to individuals? Several studies have demonstrated that using natural frequencies with a consistent denominator – the number of affected individuals per unit of population, eg three per 100,000 men – to communicate population-level risk can help to avoid misinterpretation of risk probabilities by patients and the public.[50, 63, 81] This is because natural frequencies include the reference class and indicate the baseline risk (one in 100 women, or three in 100 over-65s), elicit greater emotional imagery than more abstract statistics, and seem to correspond to the way that people intuitively think about risks.[82] When using natural frequencies, however, individuals have a tendency to assume, optimistically, that they belong to the "low risk" group.[62]

Individual risk profiles are not fixed – they change with age, risks diminish or accumulate, and vary with exposure to lifestyle risk factors. Many common diseases manifest in older age, and the risk of disease in a younger person is usually lower than for a person over 60 years of age. This is true for many cancers and dementia, among others. Using the appropriate reference class, or population, is essential for accurate and meaningful risk communication.

Reference points can also help patients and the public understand probability and absolute risk, and benchmark themselves against these reference points.[83] Including information about a threshold above or below which action should be taken, alongside absolute risk information, can aid understanding. High cholesterol is a risk factor for cardiovascular disease, for example, and the National Institute for Health and Clinical Excellence (NICE) recommends that individuals with total blood cholesterol levels above five millimoles per litre should take action to reduce their cholesterol levels, through diet and physical activity, and cholesterol-reducing drugs such as statins. Comparing a patient's absolute risk of experiencing a heart attack to that of another group without certain risk factors (eg smokers versus non-smokers), or to a familiar event (such as a car crash), can help them put their own risk into context.

A simple unit of risk can be an effective way to measure and compare different types of risk. The **micromort** describes a one in a million chance of death, and can be calculated for a range of acute risks. It is estimated, for example, that the risk of death from external causes in the UK – accidents, murders, suicides, etc – is approximately one micromort per day. One day of skiing is equivalent to half a micromort, whereas one scuba diving session is equivalent to five micromorts.[84] **Table 1** lists the risks of a range of hospital procedures in terms of micromorts. In this way, a diverse range of comparisons about the risk of death of different activities can be made, using the micromort as a standard unit.

For these comparisons to be meaningful, the relevant units of exposure (eg per day, per activity session, per 100 miles) must be clearly defined. While the micromort unit is ideal for comparisons of small, acute risks, it is not always appropriate for risks that accumulate with increased exposure. Many major public health risks fall into this category – for example the risk of death from smoking, alcohol consumption, inactivity, and high fat or sugar diets.

Table 1 – comparing the chance of death for a range of hospital events using the micromort measurement

Hospital event	Micromort
Night in hospital from avoidable causes (England and Wales)	at least 75
Caesarian operation (England and Wales)	170
Giving birth (UK)	80
Non-emergency procedure involving general anaesthesia	10

Source: adapted from Spiegelhalter and Pearson (2010),[84] Hogan (2010)[85] and Royal College of Anaesthetists (2009).[86]

2.3.4. Graphical communication

Visual information has the ability to attract and hold the viewer's attention. Information presented visually in the form of graphs has been shown to improve risk communication.[63, 87] Patients and the public process visual information more effectively than numerical information, feel that they have a clearer understanding of the information, and find visual information helpful in decision-making processes.[81, 83] It can also improve risk communication where patients have poor numeracy skills.[62]

The strength of graphics is that they can reveal patterns in complex data, and synthesise large volumes of information into a single graph or diagram.[81, 83] Features that improve the accuracy of information recall are not always the same as those that encourage behaviour change, however. The goal of the risk communication message should therefore be a consideration in graphical design.[87]

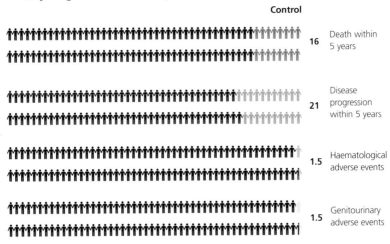

Figure 5: conventional versus adjuvant radiotherapy after surgery in early stage cervical cancer patients

Control

16 — Death within 5 years

21 — Disease progression within 5 years

1.5 — Haematological adverse events

1.5 — Genitourinary adverse events

Source: Spiegelhalter (2011) and Rogers (2009).[87, 89]

Graphical representation of information should aim to minimise the mental processing effort required to understand any dataset, include only the information relevant for understanding the issue, and can lead to higher quality decisions.[21, 88] Simplicity and clarity of design is key to achieving this. **Figure 5** illustrates the comparison between conventional treatment and adjuvant radiotherapy after surgery for patients with early stage cervical cancer.[89]

This graph compares a conventional and a new treatment option for cervical cancer, using human stick figures to visualise the differences in outcomes between treatment options, and a colour gradient to denote severity of outcome.[87]

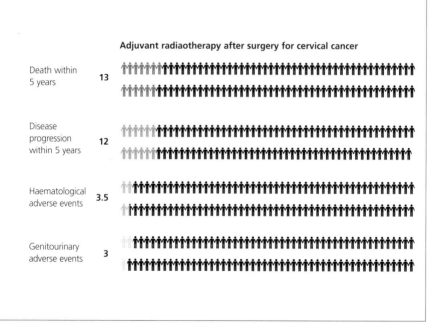

Table 2 summarises some common graphical formats that have been shown to increase patient and public understanding of risk concepts.[90]

Table 2 – Common types of graphs that can help to communicate risk concepts

Type of graph	Use
Risk ladder	Making comparisons (see Figure 9 on page 59)
Bar chart	Making comparisons (see Figure 12 on page 64)
Line graphs	Showing trends in data (see Figure 14 on page 68)
Pie charts	Judging proportions (see Figure 27 on page 120)
Scatter plots	Conveying variability in the data
Human stick figures	Showing natural frequencies, especially for low probability events (see Figure 4 on page 36-37)

Just as with verbal and numerical information, graphical information is subject to cognitive biases. Human stick figures, for example, can help avoid framing bias by showing the affected and non-affected groups in a population.[91] These graphs can invoke optimism bias, however, as viewers tend to assume they belong in the non-affected group.[87, 92] Risk ladders are useful for comparing a range of risks, but viewers are more sensitive to the position of a risk on the ladder than the actual magnitude of risk.[87]

2.3.5. Verbal communication

Doctors will invariably need to communicate risk information to patients or the public verbally. Using non-numerical descriptions of risk can help patients to put risk in perspective, but doctors should be aware that terms such as 'low risk' or 'very unlikely' will be interpreted inconsistently by different people.[21, 81, 87]

In developing the Fourth Assessment Report on Climate Change, the Intergovernmental Panel on Climate Change (IPCC) attempted to standardise the communication of information from a diverse range of scientific disciplines, and recommended that uncertainty could be communicated verbally on a scale ranging from very high confidence (>90%) through to high (>80%), medium (>50%), low (+/- 20%) or very low confidence (<10%). As with uncertainty, risk probabilities can be communicated verbally on a scale ranging from virtually certain (>99%)

through to very likely (>90%), likely (>66%), as likely as not (33 to 66%), unlikely (<33%), very unlikely (<10%) and exceptionally unlikely (<1%).[71]

Using common and known risks as a reference can improve communication and understanding of risk. Most people are aware of the risks of smoking, and an unfamiliar risk can be described with reference to these risks: the lifetime risk of developing lung cancer from average indoor exposure to radon gas in the UK is equivalent to smoking about two cigarettes per day, for example.[81, 93] For a resident of Cornwall – an area that has a high level of natural radon – the risk of lung cancer from exposure to radon gas in a poorly-ventilated home is equivalent to smoking eight cigarettes per day.[81, 93]

Reference points that individual patients can relate to aspects of their own lives – the capacity of a well-known football stadium, or the population of a local town, for example – may also aid understanding by contextualising information. Using narrative formats and stories for risk communication can increase engagement with the issue by evoking vivid, emotive imagery.[37]

2.4. Evaluating risk

When faced with risk information, what is the best way to evaluate and make decisions based on this knowledge? Individuals are often able to modify their lifestyle or environment to adjust their exposure to risks. What level of risk is acceptable to an individual or community? The answer will depend on different cultural, social and personal considerations. As a society, there is a tendency to accept lower levels of risk when the risk is involuntary (such as community exposure to a toxic chemical), and higher levels when the risk is deemed to be a matter of personal control or choice (such as smoking or alcohol consumption).[4]

Evaluating and managing risks can take place in a variety of circumstances. At the individual level, risk management can be discussed and considered as part of the patient-doctor consultation. In this context, doctors can help individual patients understand and put risk into perspective, and discuss options for patients to minimise the risks in their lives (eg providing advice to patients who are overweight about the benefits of regular physical activity).

At the population level, public health doctors and other professionals can identify and highlight particular risks affecting a population, and have an important role to play in communicating risk and helping the local population to take steps to minimise risk (eg implementing targeted vaccination programmes).

In the UK, the Health Protection Agency (HPA) is responsible for protecting the public from the health risks from infectious diseases and environmental hazards. The HPA provides information and health advice to the public, and advises health professionals, and local and national governments on these issues. The Centers for Disease Control and Prevention (CDC) is the equivalent institution in the United States. The remit of the CDC includes protecting health, the control of disease, injury and disability, and preparedness for new and emerging health risks.

2.4.1. Risk management

Risk management is the process of identifying risks, undertaking risk assessments, and implementing preventive, mitigation and control policies to reduce the level of risk, thereby minimising the incidence of harm and any knock-on effects. There are a number of strategies that can be adopted to manage risk, dependent on the nature of hazards and harms in each case, as outlined in **Table 3**.[b]

Table 3 – Examples of risk management strategies

Example of hazard/harm	Risk management strategy	Example of risk management strategy
Shattered/broken glass is frequently the cause of accidental injury or used deliberately as a weapon	Prevent the hazard from existing	The use of shatter-proof plastic containers as substitutes for pint glasses and glass bottles is common in pubs, clubs and at music festivals
Deliberate and accidental misuse of medication can lead to harmful toxic effects and death as a result of overdose	Control the use of a substance or equipment	While not all medication is prescription-only, access to many over-the-counter medications is restricted to pharmacies, in order to control their use, and misuse
Sharp objects including needles, syringes and surgical blades can cause injury and increase the risk of infection with blood borne viruses such as human Immunodeficiency virus (HIV), hepatitis B and hepatitis C	Implement safety measure to minimise exposure to a hazard	Sharps bins are a common feature in surgical settings, and are used for the safe disposal of needles, syringes and other sharp objects

---

b   As risk management is a large discipline, it will only be covered briefly here. Further information on risk management can be found from the Health and Safety Executive (HSE) and the Institute of Risk Management.

Example of hazard/harm	Risk management strategy	Example of risk management strategy
Infection with the influenza virus can cause serious illness, and in some cases, can be fatal	Develop resistance to a hazard	Immunisation against seasonal flu, via the flu vaccination offered each year, aims to prevent or ameliorate the effects of influenza infection, particularly in high-risk groups (eg older people and pregnant women)
Terrorist attacks can cause serious injury and death through unlawful use of violence (eg suicide bombings)	Mitigate the harm from a hazard	Although a future terrorist attack is not entirely preventable, an emergency preparedness plan can mitigate the potential harm, for example by ensuring a hospital has sufficient capacity to cope with a sudden influx of casualties
Individuals involved in car crashes are at a high risk of serious injury or death, predominantly as a result of high impact collisions	Modify the characteristics of a hazard so as to reduce its risk	Airbags and crash sensors are now routinely fitted to new cars, reducing the severity of impact suffered by car occupants
Exposure to asbestos increases the risk of serious illness and death from mesothelioma, lung cancer and other rarer diseases	Reduce the amount of hazard in existence	The use of asbestos as a construction material has been regulated in the UK since 1985, and its use and disposal is controlled under the Control of Asbestos Regulations 2006

Example of hazard/harm	Risk management strategy	Example of risk management strategy
Ozone depletion resulting from the release of chlorofluorocarbons (CFCs) leads to increased ultraviolet radiation and a corresponding increase in the risk of skin cancer	Prevent the release of hazard into the environment	The release of CFCs into the earth's atmosphere has been significantly reduced as a result of the introduction of the 1989 Montreal Protocol

In practice, a number of risk management strategies are used in combination to minimise the likelihood of harm from a hazard. The implementation of a ban on smoking in enclosed public spaces aims to minimise exposure to secondhand smoke, while restrictions on the sale of cigarettes aim to limit the use of tobacco in adolescents. These measures are complemented by the legislation governing the constituents of cigarettes as well as 'fire safe' regulations such as reduced ignition propensity cigarettes. The total effect contributes to diminishing the population risk of the use of cigarettes.

Within risk management, **risk assessment** is the scientific, quantitative process that aims to identify and characterise hazards and risk, as well as to assess population and individual exposure to risks. Risk assessments are often based on the type of scientific and empirical studies outlined in section 2.1.2. Uncertainty must be integrated into risk assessment and management; dealing with uncertainty is a key challenge in risk management practices (see **Box 5**, page 17).

With increasingly sensitive data collection, and growing knowledge of hazards and risk events, it is clear that risk elimination or avoidance is frequently not realistic. Residual risks will almost inevitably remain even within the most stringent risk management strategy.

The response to major disasters and emergencies is a useful way of illustrating the processes involved in risk management. Specific disaster preparedness and management strategies exist to facilitate a rapid and coordinated response to any major event. Disaster preparedness and the disaster response are aimed at intervening between the stages of progression of a disaster, with the goal of minimising its ultimate impact (see **Figure 6**). It encompasses the sum of all planning and policies implemented before the event occurs, and all organisations, from government to private and community organisations, should be involved in disaster preparedness. Risk assessment aims to identify and assess the hazards that a community may face, and establish a profile of the hazard, its probability in terms of frequency, and potential consequences in terms of human impact and property damage.

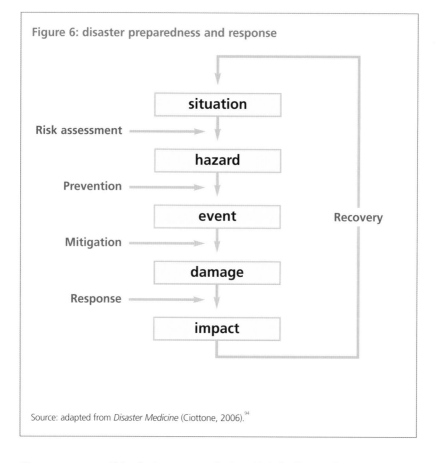

Figure 6: disaster preparedness and response

Risk assessment ⇢ situation

Prevention ⇢ hazard

Mitigation ⇢ event — Recovery

Response ⇢ damage

impact

Source: adapted from *Disaster Medicine* (Ciottone, 2006).[94]

Mitigation of damage after the event aims to prevent injury, illness and death, and to limit the loss of property. The disaster response is specific to the needs of the situation, based on the nature of the event and damage, the needs of the local population, and the geography of the area. The recovery phase aims to restore a society to its normal functioning state.

Public communication is a key element to all phases of the disaster preparedness, mitigation and response, and can help to develop and maintain public trust.[94]

An important component of risk management at a national level is consideration for the likelihood of major disasters and emergencies occurring. This allows for prioritisation of resources and effective risk management planning. In the UK, the Cabinet Office publishes a national risk register of potential civil emergencies (natural and man-made), and has classified a number of high consequence risks to the UK according to their potential impact and likelihood (see **Figure 7**). This indicates that pandemic disease, such as avian influenza, is relatively likely and potentially of serious consequence, whereas cyber attacks, although likely to occur, are not expected to have a significant impact in terms of human health or damage to infrastructure.[95]

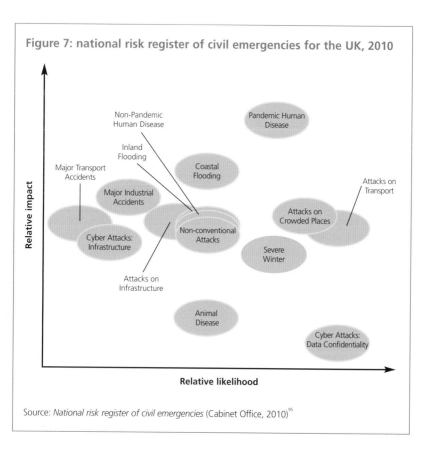

Figure 7: national risk register of civil emergencies for the UK, 2010

Relative impact

Non-Pandemic
Human Disease

Pandemic Human
Disease

Inland
Flooding

Major Transport
Accidents

Coastal
Flooding

Attacks on
Transport

Major Industrial
Accidents

Cyber Attacks:
Infrastructure

Non-conventional
Attacks

Attacks on
Crowded Places

Severe
Winter

Attacks on
Infrastructure

Animal
Disease

Cyber Attacks:
Data Confidentiality

Relative likelihood

Source: *National risk register of civil emergencies* (Cabinet Office, 2010)[95]

Vulnerability to a disaster is dependent on susceptibility and resilience of the population and the environment. Poverty is the most important risk factor for vulnerability to a disaster. **Susceptibility** to a disaster can be affected by the local geography and environment, but also by protection measures that strengthen defences against the disaster, such as earthquake building codes, backup generators, and protection of key utilities. **Resilience** is the capability of the population or the environment to cope with the event, by adapting to, buffering or absorbing the effects. Disaster preparedness can improve the resilience of a society to a disaster, thereby reducing its vulnerability.[94]

2.4.2. Risk evaluation

The risk evaluation process seeks to prioritise risk management strategies and consider the wider social, cultural and political context surrounding risks and hazards. This helps to determine whether and to what extent a particular risk deserves attention and resources.[4]

Risk management unavoidably faces compromise, competing interests, and financial restrictions. A tension that arises frequently is the fine balance between the motivation to maximise safety and the need to preserve personal freedom of choice. These tensions are frequently highlighted in debates surrounding road safety measures, restrictions on food composition or ingredients, or access to tobacco and alcohol products. Speed cameras are very effective at reducing traffic speed and collisions on dangerous roads;[96] but there is considerable public opposition to their use because of the perceived restrictions to freedom of movement, high cost, and use of revenue. Some people argue that if the acceptable threshold of risk is set too low this will diminish rather than enhance the overall level of safety because it will discredit the concept of 'risk management' and 'health and safety'. They fear it would disable people's normal capacities for risk management, overwhelming them with a set of tasks which are impossible to achieve in total and may not be prioritised appropriately.[97]

Medical information relating to health risks contributes to risk evaluation judgements, typically at the risk assessment stage. This scientific evidence is only one component of any risk evaluation process, and is not necessarily the most important factor in every instance. Risk evaluation rarely considers risk alone and often transforms itself into an opportunity for individuals and communities to discuss the wider social and political context of any given issue.[4] Experience and scientific information can complement each other and lead to better risk evaluation outcomes.[4]

In the UK, the HSE developed and adopted a 'tolerability of risk' framework as an outcome of the public inquiry into the Sizewell B Nuclear Power Station in 1988.[98] This framework sets basic safety limits and general levels of unacceptable risk to workers and the general population. The HSE determined that a risk was broadly acceptable when the annual risk of death was one in 1,000,000 or less. A risk was considered unacceptable when the annual risk of death was one in 10,000 or more.

Risks that fell between one in 1,000,000 and one in 10,000 were deemed to be tolerable, but responsible parties have a duty to minimise and maintain these risks to a level as low as reasonably practicable (commonly referred to as 'ALARP') (see **Figure 8**).[98]

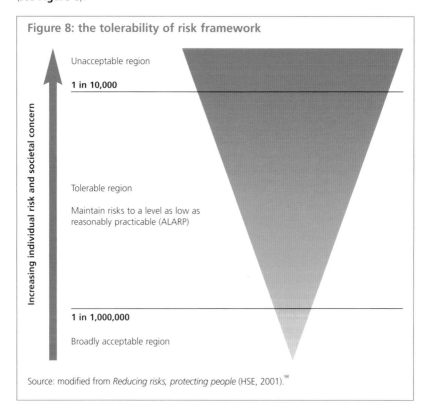

Figure 8: the tolerability of risk framework

Increasing individual risk and societal concern

Unacceptable region

1 in 10,000

Tolerable region

Maintain risks to a level as low as reasonably practicable (ALARP)

1 in 1,000,000

Broadly acceptable region

Source: modified from *Reducing risks, protecting people* (HSE, 2001).[98]

Evaluating and acting on health risks involves more than just applying medical knowledge to achieve the minimum possible level of risk. Medical and scientific information typically feed into risk evaluation processes in the form of risk assessment. Individual, social and cultural values have an important role to play, and can be harnessed through public engagement.

2.4.3. The precautionary principle

It is not always possible to gather sufficient data on cause and effect, and adequately characterise new or unknown risks within the timeframe needed for decision-making. The concept of the **precautionary principle** was developed to address this issue.[4] Where there is a high level of uncertainty surrounding risk cause, escalation or consequence, it is prudent to attempt to minimise the potential for harm, without making decisions that are irreversible.

The precautionary principle was developed in Germany in the 1970s as part of a broader environmental philosophy in response to emerging environmental risks such as acid rain, pollution in the North Sea, and climate change. It was subsequently included in the Maastricht Treaty of 1991, governing membership of the EU, and has been invoked in a number of decisions by the European Court of Justice – including in relation to trade restrictions on US beef treated with hormones, genetically-modified foodstuffs, and restrictions on the export of beef from the UK during the BSE crisis in 1998.[99]

There is no formal definition of the precautionary principle, nor a recommended implementation strategy. The 1998 Wingspread international conference on the precautionary principle defined it as:

> When an activity raises threats of harm to human health or the environment, precautionary measures should be taken even if some cause and effect relationships are not fully established scientifically.[100]

This approach to managing uncertainty can be very effective but has a number of weaknesses. Determining an acceptable level of risk and the proportionality of response based on limited and uncertain information is inherently difficult. It can lead to unnecessarily strict regulations being implemented and erring on the side of caution, which might waste resources or have significant cost implications. When information on a risk is sparse, recognition of leadership and expertise on the topic can be in dispute, and risk evaluation is open to interpretation from interested parties, such as in debates surrounding the environmental and health risks of climate change (see **Box 7**).

Box 7 – precautionary principle and climate change mitigation
Climate change science involves understanding of the interaction of a number of complex systems – atmosphere, ecosystems, human activity, etc – and necessarily involves a high degree of uncertainty, in particular in predicting the impacts of a range of future scenarios.

The precautionary principle can be applied to address the risks of climate change, against a background of inherent uncertainty, the complexity of climate science, ongoing research, and the potential for harm. Unusually for the precautionary principle, it is the status quo that poses a threat to the environment and human health, in the form of rising greenhouse gas emissions and increasing global average temperatures.[100]

A precautionary approach would therefore recommend action to mitigate the risks of climate change through measures to minimise or offset greenhouse gas emissions. The 1992 UN Framework Convention on Climate Change (UNFCCC) takes this view and states that:

> *"The Parties should take precautionary measures to anticipate, prevent or minimise the causes of climate change and mitigate its adverse effects. Where there are threats of serious or irreversible damage, lack of full scientific certainty should not be used as a reason for postponing such measures, taking into account that policies and measures to deal with climate change should be cost effective so as to ensure global benefits at the lowest possible cost (Article 3.3)."*[101]

Similarly, Principle 15 of the 1992 Rio Declaration on Environment and Development states that:

> *"In order to protect the environment, the precautionary approach shall be widely applied by States according to their capabilities. Where there are threats of serious or irreversible damage, lack of full scientific certainty shall not be used as a reason for postponing cost-effective measures to prevent environmental degradation."*[102]

2.4.4.   The dual use dilemma

A dilemma arises when scientific research or technologies intended to benefit public good can also be misused. The development of new drugs are intended to benefit people but some could also be used as bioweapons. In these instances, scientists and others are presented with the problem of how to prevent misuse without foregoing any beneficial application or limiting scientific progress. This is becoming increasingly important with the rapid pace of technological and scientific development – including recent advances in genome sequencing, synthetic biology, nanotechnology and bioinformatics – and the difficulty in predicting future applications of new technologies.[103-105]

There are a number of examples of the **dual use dilemma** in the biosciences. The 2004 BMA Board of Science report *Biotechnology, weapons and humanity* warned of the potential misuse of microbial pathogens (eg bacteria and viruses) and bioregulators that could disrupt cellular processes or organ systems (eg neurotransmitters, endorphins, cytokines). In the aftermath of the 2001 terrorist attacks on the World Trade Centre in New York City, scientists at the University of New York in Stonybrook demonstrated that it was possible to reconstruct the poliovirus from fragments of DNA purchased over the internet. They said they "made the virus to send a warning that terrorists might be able to make biological weapons without obtaining a natural virus".[106] A similar study in 2005 demonstrated that the 1918 human influenza virus could be reconstructed using synthetic biology techniques.[107] These developments demonstrated the power of a technology that could be used to promote human wellbeing, or malignantly to produce harm. Debate continues over the value of the research and its publications, and solutions to reduce the risk are still lacking.

The Research Councils, Wellcome Trust, and the Society of Microbiology have developed policies on codes of conduct and the misuse of science. The major scientific journals Science, Nature and Proceedings of the National Academy of Sciences, alongside the American Society of Microbiology, signed a joint statement on scientific publication and security, stating that when "harm of publication outweighs the potential societal benefits… the paper should be modified or not published".

The UK House of Commons Science and Technology Committee published a report on science and terrorism in 2003, and recommended that scientists engaging in research with the potential for dual use should subscribe to an ethical code of conduct.[108] Other measures that might be necessary, depending on the threat, are limiting the scope of research on a particular topic, or access to necessary equipment. A similar approach has been adopted by scientific and research organisations across the world, and in the US, led to the establishment of a National Science Advisory Board on Biosecurity (NSABB), which provides "advice, guidance and leadership" on dual use research.

LIVING WITH RISKS TO HEALTH

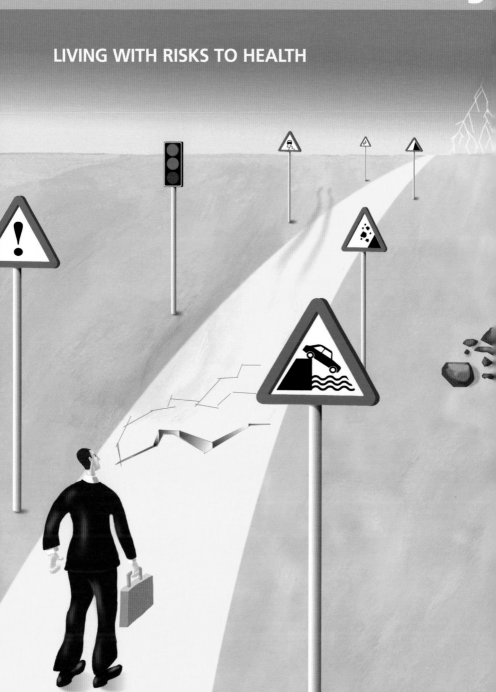

3. LIVING WITH RISKS TO HEALTH

3.1. Risk in perspective

Nothing in life is free from risk – risk is simply impossible to avoid. There are a near infinite number of factors and circumstances that can influence an individual's risk of death or disease, from the extremely rare to the everyday.

One might judge, for example, that it is safer to stay at home in bed rather than venture out into the world and risk being hit by a car, injured playing sports, or struck by lightning. But staying at home presents other, different risks – accidents, fire, and poisoning are common risks in the home, as are the consequences of a lifetime of staying inactive indoors. Even ordinary activities – eating breakfast, watching television, walking the dog – carry risks, however minor.

A sound understanding of the major risks to health, their relative magnitudes, and knowledge of risk factors, cause and consequences, can help put risk into context. Doctors, as key communicators of health information, should have a good understanding of these concepts.

The important question is: what are the greatest risks to health? In other words, what are the most common, and the most likely, causes of death, disability and loss of quality of life? What are the major risk factors that increase the likelihood of death by these causes? How do these absolute risks relate to the public perception – are they exaggerated or disregarded? Keeping these questions in mind will help to maintain perspective.

The risk ladder presented in **Figure 9** is one way of visualising and comparing the diverse health risks individuals may face – from the major to the extremely remote – and is based on the most recent UK data. The aim is to put risk into perspective, by visualising a range of common and perceived risks together. While this is an approximation and oversimplification of the risk to an individual – individuals are not all at equal risk due to differences in social determinants, lifestyle, environment and genetic makeup – it is included to provide an idea of the key health risks in their relative order of magnitude. At a glance, there is a significantly greater risk of dying from cardiovascular disease than MRSA, of dementia than homicide, although public perceptions of risk do not necessarily reflect this.

Figure 9: a risk ladder of the common risks of death per 100,000 population in the UK

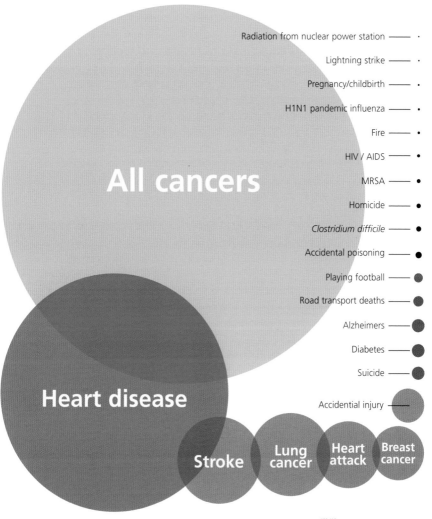

All cancers

Heart disease

Stroke

Lung cancer

Heart attack

Breast cancer

Radiation from nuclear power station — ·
Lightning strike — ·
Pregnancy/childbirth — ·
H1N1 pandemic influenza — ·
Fire — ·
HIV / AIDS — •
MRSA — •
Homicide — •
Clostridium difficile — •
Accidental poisoning — ●
Playing football — ●
Road transport deaths — ●
Alzheimers — ●
Diabetes — ●
Suicide — ●
Accidental injury — ●

Source: modified from *Mortality statistics* (ONS, 2010) and Calman (1996)[109-110]

This chapter explores the major health risks and their main risk factors. For each, it provides an overview of the hazards, harm, risk and risk factors, and evidence of how common the health risk is in the UK. Interspersed within this mainly factual information are discussion sections that aim to illustrate the risk concepts introduced in chapter 2.

3.1.1. What are the greatest risks to health and wellbeing?

There remain stark contrasts in the global burden of diseases between developing and developed countries – in terms of the variation in mortality rates, the age distribution of mortality, the total numbers of people affected, and the types of diseases they suffer. Globally, it is cardiovascular disease – CHD, stroke and cerebrovascular disease – that is the leading cause of death. Infectious diseases remain the leading causes of death in low income developing countries, with cardiovascular and childhood diseases also significant contributors to mortality. Non-communicable diseases including cardiovascular diseases and cancer have replaced infectious diseases as the leading causes of death in high income developed countries like the UK.

Many middle income countries are experiencing an epidemiological transition, and suffer a double burden of the diseases of low and high income countries. Non-communicable diseases are becoming more prevalent, but infectious diseases are not yet under control, leaving these countries with a wide spectrum of disease and placing extreme strain on health systems and resources.[111, 112-114]

What factors influence an individual's risk of death from these diseases? Data on the key risk factors that contribute to the global burden of disease have been compiled by the WHO (see **Figures 10** and **11**). The most recent available data show that these too vary greatly between low, middle and high income countries. Globally, risk factors associated with high income lifestyles are overtaking poverty-related risk factors in their contribution to global mortality. Unsafe sex is also a major health risk factor because of its role in the HIV/AIDS epidemic.[111, 115]

In high income countries, the major health risks are overwhelmingly lifestyle factors such as tobacco and alcohol use, high blood pressure, high cholesterol, high glucose, overweight, and physical inactivity. In low income developing countries, underweight, unsafe sex, unsafe water and poor sanitation, and nutritional deficiencies are the major health risk factors. Tobacco, high cholesterol, high blood pressure and high blood glucose also contribute significantly to the burden of disease in these countries. As with the causes of mortality, middle income countries are exposed to the risk factors prevalent in high and low income countries.[115]

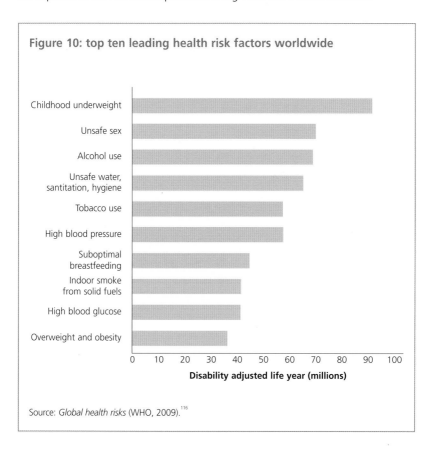

Figure 10: top ten leading health risk factors worldwide

Source: *Global health risks* (WHO, 2009).[116]

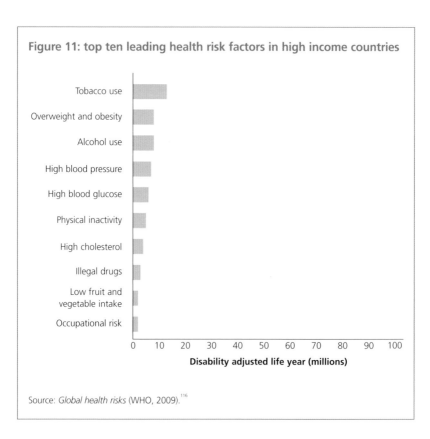

Figure 11: top ten leading health risk factors in high income countries

Tobacco use
Overweight and obesity
Alcohol use
High blood pressure
High blood glucose
Physical inactivity
High cholesterol
Illegal drugs
Low fruit and vegetable intake
Occupational risk

0   10   20   30   40   50   60   70   80   90   100

Disability adjusted life year (millions)

Source: *Global health risks* (WHO, 2009).[116]

As outlined in the 2009 BMA Board of Science report *Early life nutrition and lifelong health*, nutritional status emerges as a key risk factor for health status – whether from undernourishment and nutrient deprivation in low income countries, or from overweight, high blood pressure, cholesterol and blood glucose in all countries.

The following sections take a closer look at the key risk factors and the major causes of death in the UK, from everyday lifestyle and medical risks, to healthcare and environmental health risks.

3.2. Everyday lifestyle risks

In the course of everyday life, individuals are exposed to a range of hazards that increase their risk of illness or death. Individuals may be able to exercise some degree of personal control over the lifestyle risk factors, such as tobacco, alcohol and drug use, physical inactivity and unsafe sex. Socioeconomic status, occupation, age and gender can also influence exposure to hazards.

3.2.1. Tobacco use

Tobacco use is a major lifestyle risk factor for ill health, and is the leading preventable cause of death in the UK. It is the leading cause of mortality and morbidity in the developed world, and the fourth leading cause globally. Tobacco is estimated to account for 17 per cent of the burden of disease in the UK,[117] and four per cent worldwide.[116]

Most people are aware that smoking causes lung cancer. This fact has been rigorously established and repeatedly demonstrated over decades of medical research. Research has shown that carcinogens in tobacco smoke also cause cancers of the lower urinary tract, pancreas, stomach, liver, other respiratory and digestive tract cancers (oral cavity, pharynx, larynx, nasal cavity, oesophagus and stomach), and myeloid leukaemia.[7, 112, 116-119] Awareness of the link between tobacco and lung cancer is very high, but smoking remains a significant public health concern.

The public is less aware that tobacco smoking causes significantly more deaths from cardiovascular and respiratory diseases than it does from cancer.[118] This includes chronic obstructive pulmonary disease (COPD), ischaemic heart disease, cerebrovascular diseases (including stroke), and rarer respiratory and cardiovascular diseases. Passive smoking – exposure to cigarette smoke and exhaled smoke – also poses a significant health risk, especially to children living with smoking parents or relatives.[6, 111, 113, 116]

Even very low levels of tobacco smoking increase the risk of cancer, respiratory and cardiovascular disease. The more cigarettes an individual smokes per day, the greater their risk of premature death from all causes (see **Figure 12**).[7] Risk of death from tobacco use also increases exponentially as smokers age.[7]

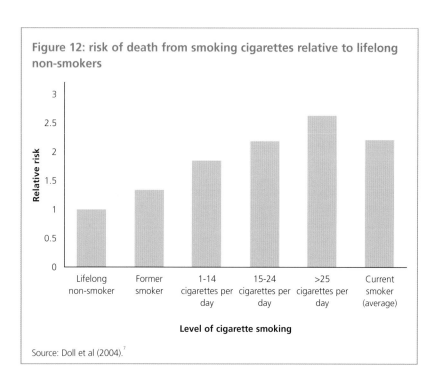

Figure 12: risk of death from smoking cigarettes relative to lifelong non-smokers

Relative risk

Level of cigarette smoking

Source: Doll et al (2004).[7]

How significant are the risks from smoking in the UK?

Smoking remains a major public health issue in the UK, despite the reduction in smoking prevalence since its height in the mid-20th century. The BMA Board of Science has reviewed the impact of smoking on health in several reports, including *Smoking and reproductive life* (2004), *Breaking the cycle of children's exposure to tobacco smoke* (2007), and most recently *Forever Cool: the influence of smoking imagery on young people* (2008).

Approximately 21 per cent of men and 20 per cent of women are regular smokers, compared to 42 and 36 per cent in 1980, respectively.[117] A socioeconomic gradient exists in smoking prevalence, with smoking more common in routine and manual labourer socioeconomic groups than in managerial and professional groups (see **Figure 13**).[122]

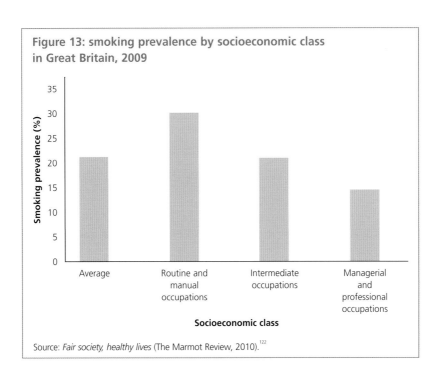

Figure 13: smoking prevalence by socioeconomic class in Great Britain, 2009

Smoking prevalence (%)

Average | Routine and manual occupations | Intermediate occupations | Managerial and professional occupations

Socioeconomic class

Source: *Fair society, healthy lives* (The Marmot Review, 2010).[122]

This smoking prevalence translates into an increased risk of premature death in the UK. The Department of Health (DH) estimates that 17 per cent of all deaths in England in 2009 – more than 82,000 deaths – could be attributed to smoking.[117] The death rate due to smoking for people over 35 years of age in the UK has been calculated at 213.2 people per 100,000 population.[117]

Summary
Tobacco use is widely recognised as the greatest preventable health risk. Despite a high level of public awareness of the harms of tobacco use, smoking remains a major public health issue in the UK.

3.2.2.   Alcohol consumption

Alcohol consumption is a significant health risk factor in the UK and globally.
The scale of alcohol consumption and its widespread use in the UK means that
it has a major impact on health.

Alcohol consumption poses immediate and long-term chronic risks to health, along
with wider social harms. Alcohol remains a significant cause of mortality and
morbidity across Europe and globally. It is the fifth leading contributor to the global
burden of disease, and estimated to account for 6.5 per cent of the burden of
disease in Europe, and four per cent worldwide.[112]

The acute direct and indirect health harms from alcohol include intoxication,
alcohol poisoning, unsafe sex, and injuries – including violence and assault, falls,
fire, drowning, road traffic crashes and occupational injuries.[126-129] Chronic alcohol
consumption can cause alcohol dependence, liver cirrhosis, alcoholic psychoses,
alcoholic cardiomyopathy, polyneuropathy and gastritis.[126] Chronic alcohol
consumption is also a risk factor for and contributory cause of hypertension,
cardiac arrhythmia, stroke, depression, epilepsy, acute and chronic pancreatitis,
gastro-oesophageal haemorrhage, and several cancers (liver, breast, lip,
oesophageal, oropharangeal, and laryngeal).[126] The health impacts of alcohol
consumption are further reviewed in the BMA Board of Science report *Alcohol
misuse: tackling the UK epidemic* (2008).[126]

Unlike tobacco, where there is no threshold level of consumption below which harm does not occur, moderate alcohol consumption may not necessarily lead to significant chronic ill health, and may have modest health benefits in certain age groups.[127-128, 130] In the UK population, the harms of alcohol consumption far outweigh the modest benefits to health. A dose-response relationship exists with alcohol consumption where, above one drink per day (approximately 2-3 units), increased consumption is directly related to increased risk of premature death, cancer, and cerebrovascular disease (see **Figure 14**).[126, 130] Alcohol consumption also significantly increases the risk of CHD: the risk is more than six times greater in heavy drinkers (more than 6 per day) than in non-drinkers.[130] This dose-response effect led to the introduction of recommended drinking guidelines[c] in the UK in 1987.

---

c   Recommended drinking guidelines are set by the UK Government to provide advice on daily and weekly maximum alcohol consumption levels – commonly referred to as "sensible drinking guidelines". The guidelines recommend that men should not regularly drink more than three to four units of alcohol per day, women should not regularly drink more than two to three units of alcohol per day, and men and women should not drink on every day of the week. In terms of weekly limits, men are advised to drink no more than 21 units per week and women no more than 14 units per week. These guidelines are currently under review.

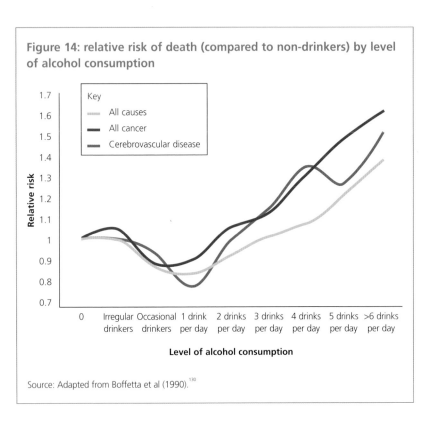

Figure 14: relative risk of death (compared to non-drinkers) by level of alcohol consumption

Key
- All causes
- All cancer
- Cerebrovascular disease

Source: Adapted from Boffetta et al (1990).[130]

How serious is the health risk from alcohol consumption in the UK?
Alcohol is having a significant impact on the health of the UK population. Its consumption has increased steadily in the UK over the past 60 years (see **Figure 15**) for all types of alcoholic beverages, and in particular for wine and spirits, which have higher alcohol content by volume.[126] A snapshot of alcohol consumption in 2009 found that the average weekly alcohol consumption was 16.8 units for men and 8.6 units for women, but 21 per cent of men and 14 per cent of women also reported binge drinking (drinking more than 8 or 6 units of alcohol in one day respectively).[131]

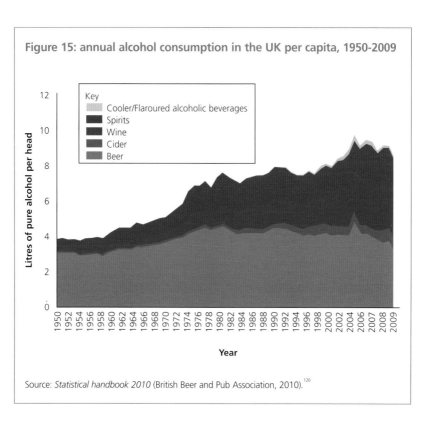

Figure 15: annual alcohol consumption in the UK per capita, 1950-2009

Key
▨ Cooler/Flaroured alcoholic beverages
■ Spirits
■ Wine
■ Cider
■ Beer

Litres of pure alcohol per head

Year

Source: *Statistical handbook 2010* (British Beer and Pub Association, 2010).[126]

Deaths directly attributable to alcohol have doubled in the UK since 1992, from 6.7 per 100,000 population in 1992 to 12.8 per 100,000 in 2009. This translates to 4,023 deaths in 1992, rising to 9,031 deaths in 2008, and 8,664 in 2009. This risk is higher for men than for women, and greatest in older adults (55 to 74 years old).[132-133]

These figures are conservative and do not include the significant number of deaths where alcohol is a contributing factor, including cardiovascular disease and stroke. Road traffic crashes to which drink driving contribute are not accounted for in these mortality data. In 2010, there were nearly 6,630 road traffic casualties as a result of driving above the legal alcohol limit, and in which 250 people were estimated to be killed and 1,230 seriously injured.[135] Although these figures are decreasing from high levels in the 1970s, they still represent 17 per cent of all road fatalities and five per cent of all serious road traffic injuries.[135]

Risk perception and alcohol consumption

Although the adverse health effects of alcohol consumption are widely recognised, public awareness and understanding of recommended drinking guidelines is lower. In a 2009 NHS Information Centre survey, more than 90 per cent of respondents correctly identified a number of health risks directly associated with alcohol consumption, including the risk of accidents, alcohol poisoning and liver disease.[136] The majority also recognised a link between alcohol consumption and the risk of depression, CHD, hypertension, stroke and pancreatitis.[136]

Awareness of the existence of recommended drinking guidelines is also growing. Knowledge of what constitutes 'sensible' drinking is mixed, however, in part due to confusion surrounding the relationship between a drink measure and an alcoholic 'unit', and the revision of the drinking guidelines.[126, 137] Even among those who are aware of recommended drinking guidelines, very few monitor their own alcohol consumption on a daily or weekly basis.[136] Alcohol content is not always marked on bottles, cans, and menus, making awareness of units more difficult. Optimism bias may lead many people to underestimate their risk of ill-health based on their own drinking habits, and less likely to monitor and moderate their alcohol consumption.

Summary

Alcohol consumption is a risk factor for a number of illnesses and injuries. Despite its modest health benefits, alcohol consumption causes significant harm in the UK. Public perception of the risks of alcohol consumption underestimates the health risk.

Further BMA resources:
- *Under the influence – the damaging effect of alcohol marketing on young people.* British Medical Association (2009).[138]
- *Alcohol misuse: tackling the UK epidemic.* British Medical Association (2008).[126]
- *Fetal alcohol spectrum disorders.* British Medical Association (2007).[139]

3.2.3. Drug use[d]

Tobacco and alcohol are arguably the psychoactive drugs that pose the most significant health risks in the UK and globally. This is partially due to their major impacts on health and wellbeing, but also because of their widespread use. Use of other recreational psychoactive drugs has a proportionally smaller impact on population health – accounting for only 0.8 per cent of global, and 2 per cent of the European burden of disease – in part due to their uncommon use in the general population.[112, 115-116]

Psychoactive drugs pose significant health risks to users and the wider community. This category of drug includes many of the illegal drugs such as heroin, cocaine and crack cocaine, barbiturates, methadone, ketamine, benzodiazepines, amphetamines, cannabis, Lysergic acid diethylamide (LSD) and ecstasy. The cultural and social attitudes surrounding illegal drugs mean that their classification and legal status do not directly relate to the health risks they pose to users and communities.[140]

Illegal drugs can have a number of acute and chronic effects on the human body, ranging from the fatal to the relatively harmless. These include overdose and fatal poisoning, addiction, heart attack, viral infection, psychosis and other mental disorders, hallucination, and the effects of intoxication, dependence and withdrawal.[120] Drug harms are not limited to the drug user – they can also cause social harms in the form of damage to family and social relationships, as well as increased costs to healthcare, social care, police and judicial systems.[140] The route

---

d   The BMA Board of Science is currently undertaking a project examining the role of the medical profession in tackling drugs of dependence.

of administration of a drug is an important factor in its risk of harm. Drugs that are injected intravenously – such as heroin – carry a high risk of fatal overdose and infection from blood borne viruses such as HIV and hepatitis.

In a 2007 study, experts in the UK – psychologists, police, pharmacologists, epidemiologists, forensic scientists – were asked to assess a range of psychoactive drugs on a scale of physical and social harms. The five most harmful drugs were determined to be heroin, cocaine, barbiturates, (street) methadone, and alcohol.[120] In a 2010 update of the study, alcohol was classified as the most harmful drug, with heroin and crack cocaine in second and third place, respectively.[140] Also in 2010, a Dutch addiction medicine expert group conducted a risk assessment of 19 recreational drugs (17 illegal drugs plus alcohol and tobacco), and ranked them on the basis of acute and chronic toxicity, addictive potency, and social harm.[141] The study ranked alcohol, tobacco, heroin, crack cocaine, and methamphetamine as being most harmful, with benzodiazepines, gamma-Hydroxybutyric acid (GHB), cannabis, ecstasy and ketamine scoring in the moderately harmful range. Magic mushrooms, LSD and khat were regarded as the least harmful of the drugs in the study.

How serious are the health risks from drug use in the UK?
Data from various surveys show that drug use is common and rare; common in the sense that over one third of the population has ever used an illegal drug in their lifetime (36.2 per cent of 16 to 59 year olds in the UK in 2008/09); rare in the sense that few (10.0%) have used drugs in the last year (recent use), and even fewer (5.8%) are current drug users.[142] Drug use among young people under the age of 16 broadly mirrors that of the UK adult population, with 15 per cent of 11 to 15 year old pupils reporting taking drugs in the last year, and seven per cent current use.[143]

There is huge variation in the types of drugs used, the demographics of users as well as geographical differences. Cannabis is the most commonly used drug across all recall periods, followed by cocaine powder, ecstasy and amphetamines for recent and current use.[142]

In 2010, there were 1,784 deaths due to drug use or poisoning in England and Wales, of whom three quarters were male (see **Figure 16**). Since 1993, the first year in which these statistics were collected, deaths have more than doubled for men and increased by almost 50 per cent for women.[144] The majority of these deaths are due to class A drug use, in particular heroin, morphine, methadone and cocaine.[144] This number also includes medically licensed drugs such as paracetamol (9%) and antidepressants (14%). Drug misuse amounts to approximately 6.8 deaths per 100,000 population in England for men, and three for women.[144]

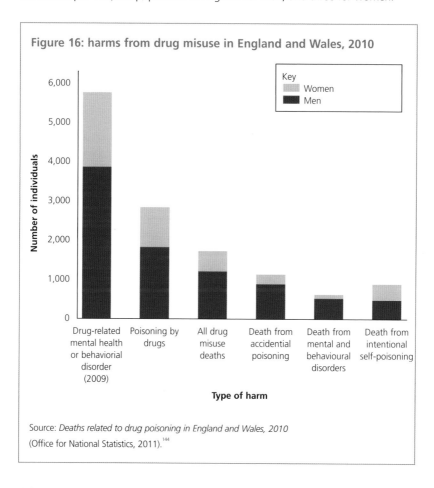

Figure 16: harms from drug misuse in England and Wales, 2010

Source: *Deaths related to drug poisoning in England and Wales, 2010* (Office for National Statistics, 2011).[144]

Injecting drug users are also at secondary risk of viral infection and systemic sepsis. More than one third of injecting drug users share needles, syringes and other equipment used to prepare drugs, and four in five engage in unsafe sex. Prevalence of HIV among injecting drug users is stable at 1.5 per cent, according to Health Protection Agency (HPA) data. Hepatitis B prevalence is decreasing due to uptake of the hepatitis B vaccine. The reverse is true for hepatitis C prevalence, which has increased since the 1990s to its current level of 47 per cent of injecting drug users.[145]

Summary

The risk associated with drug use varies according to the drug. For drugs such as heroin, crack cocaine, the risk of harm to drug users and the communities in which they live can be high. Because drug use is relatively uncommon, compared to tobacco and alcohol use, the burden of harm to the population is lower.

3.2.4.   Unsafe sex

Unsafe sex (sexual activity in which precautions are not taken to reduce the risk of acquiring or spreading disease) and sexually-transmitted infections (STIs) are a major contributor to the global burden of disease, predominantly due to the effect of the HIV epidemic in low income developing countries.[111] Ninety-nine per cent of HIV infection was attributed to unsafe sex in African countries.[115] In high and middle income countries, the health burden of unsafe sex is significantly lower, as is HIV prevalence, but it remains an important cause of disease and mortality. Mortality from cervical cancer, as a result of human papilloma virus (HPV) infection, accounts for 11 per cent of deaths attributed to unsafe sex worldwide.[111]

Sexually transmitted infections are viral or bacterial infections that are transmitted by person to person sexual contact. Some can also be transmitted from mother to child during pregnancy, birth or breastfeeding. Common STIs include gonorrhoea, chlamydia, genital herpes, genital warts, hepatitis B, syphilis and HIV. Infections can have serious health consequences including infertility, ectopic pregnancy, cervical cancer and premature death in those infected, and in infants infected through maternal contact.

Unsafe sex in the UK

Sexually transmitted infections have become more prevalent among the UK population in the past ten years. As highlighted in the 2002 BMA Board of Science report *Sexually transmitted infections*, the risk of STI infection is not evenly distributed in the population. Diagnoses are highly concentrated among young people in the 16 to 24 age group, however the number of people aged over 45 diagnosed with an STI is also increasing. The prevalence of common STIs in the general population in 2010 is estimated to be:

• Chlamydia: 348.8 per 100,000 population
• Gonorrhoea: 30.1 per 100,000 population.[146]

The number of people infected with HIV in the UK is increasing; new infections are slightly declining. In 2009, an estimated 86,500 people were living with HIV – 173 per 100,000 adults aged 15-59 – where approximately 26 per cent were unaware of their infection.[147] There were 6,630 new HIV diagnoses in 2009, of which nearly half were likely to have been acquired within the UK.[147]

Summary

While public awareness of unsafe sex as a risk factor for acquiring a STI is high in the UK, in particular in relation to HIV infection, unsafe sex and the prevalence of STIs are increasing.

Further BMA resources:

• *Sexual health clinics – examples of good practice.* British Medical Association (2006).[148]
• *Sexually transmitted infection, update.* British Medical Association (2008).[149]

3.2.5. Overweight and obesity

Overweight and obesity are one of the more apparent effects of the modern lifestyles common in the developed world. These conditions occur as a result of the excess accumulation of body fat, and can be defined as having a body mass index (BMI) of between 25 and 30 kg/m^2 (overweight), and 30 kg/m^2 or more (obese).

Both conditions can lead to premature death. They are also risk factors for cardiovascular disease, diabetes, hypertension, certain cancers (breast, colon and endometrial) and musculoskeletal disorders such as osteoarthritis.[150] A dose-response relationship has been observed, where risk of disease has been shown to increase steadily from a BMI of 25 upwards.[151-152] Body fat distribution appears to be an important predictor of disease risk, with visceral fat and increased waist circumference particularly associated with a higher risk.[153]

The BMA Board of Science report *Preventing childhood obesity* (2005)[154] provides a more extensive review of the health impacts of overweight and obesity and addresses how to tackle the risk factors for obesity. This report, together with the BMA Board of Science *Early life nutrition and lifelong health* (2009)[155] report, which discusses the impact of maternal diet and breastfeeding on childhood obesity, are discussed further in section 3.2.8.

In their simplest form, overweight and obesity are a result of energy imbalance in the body, where the amount of energy consumed as food (calories) outweighs the amount of energy expended. The reasons for this imbalance are multifaceted and influenced by changing diets, culture, social norms, surrounding environment, and genetics.[153] The 20th century saw a shift in diet towards processed and energy-dense foods rich in fat and sugar and low in micronutrients, and a trend towards less physical activity and more sedentary lifestyles, work patterns and transportation modes. This combination of factors has been classified as an 'obesogenic environment' – an environment that increases the risk of overweight and obesity.[153]

Alongside the obesogenic environment, many people are unaware of the health impacts of overweight and obesity, and have an inaccurate perception of their own body weight.[156] This lack of knowledge and 'optimism bias' leads individuals to underestimate their health risks associated with their body weight.

How serious is the health risk from overweight and obesity?
Overweight and obesity are a major public health concern globally, accounting for two per cent of global and seven per cent of the disease burden in high income countries. The WHO estimates that by 2015, 2.3 billion adults will be overweight and 700 million obese worldwide.[111]

In 2010, approximately 66 per cent of men and 57 per cent of women in England were overweight or obese (with a BMI over 25 kg/m^2), and almost one quarter of men and women were obese (with a BMI over 30 kg/m^2).[156] At the same time, 20 to 25 per cent of children were estimated to be overweight.[156] In 1980, only six per cent of men and eight per cent of women in England were obese.[156] With no sign of a change in the obesogenic environment in the UK, a Government Office for Science Foresight report on obesity predicted that approximately 40 per cent of the population will be obese by 2025, rising to 50 per cent in 2050.[153]

Taking into account an individual's waist circumference, this increase in body weight means that 19 per cent of men are estimated to be at increased risk, 14 per cent at high risk and 20 per cent at very high risk of developing long-term health problems, as defined by NICE.[132] For women, these figures are 14, 18 and 23 per cent respectively. Obesity is responsible for 9,000 premature deaths a year in England, and in 2008, 24 per cent of men and 25 per cent of women were obese (see **Figure 17**).[117, 156]

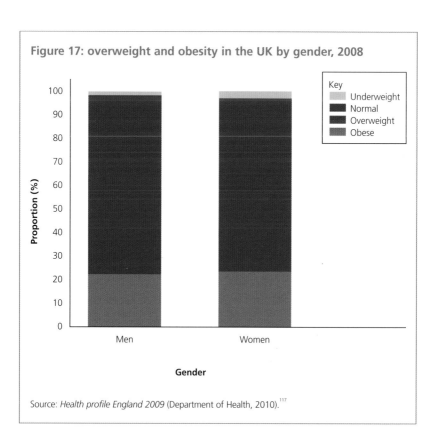

Figure 17: overweight and obesity in the UK by gender, 2008

Key
Underweight
Normal
Overweight
Obese

Proportion (%)

Men   Women

Gender

Source: *Health profile England 2009* (Department of Health, 2010).[117]

Summary

Overweight and obesity are risk factors for cardiovascular disease, diabetes, hypertension, certain cancers, musculoskeletal disorders, and premature death. These health harms associated with overweight and obesity are under-recognised by the public, and obesity is on the rise in the UK.

Further BMA resources:
• *Preventing childhood obesity.* British Medical Association (2005).[154]

3.2.6. Physical inactivity

Physical inactivity is a widespread feature of modern life. Over the past century, work and transportation patterns have shifted towards more sedentary forms. For the most part physical activity has not been displaced to leisure time – this, too, is dominated by sedentary activities.

Physical inactivity is not simply a lack of exercise; it comprises a set of sedentary activities that require very low levels of energy. Sedentary activity in itself is a risk factor for conditions such as cardiovascular disease and obesity, independent of a lack of physical exercise, which also increases these risks.[153, 157]

Regular physical activity is a protective factor and reduces the risk of a range of conditions such as obesity, diabetes, hypertension, CHD, stroke and mental illness.[156-158] Physical activity is not only a means of weight loss – these protective effects are observed irrespective of an individual's BMI or weight loss.[153] The UK-wide Chief Medical Officers (CMOs) have developed separate guidelines aimed at the early years, children and young people, adults and older adults, to encourage physical activity across the life course.[157] The BMA has recognised the many health benefits of common physical activities such as walking and cycling in a number of Board of Science reports, including *Road transport and health* (1997), *Preventing childhood obesity* (2005) and *Transport and health* (2009).

Physical activity levels are very low in the UK and have been declining for the past 30 years.[156] At the same time, sedentary activity is increasing, with one third of men and women sedentary for six or more hours on weekdays, and watching on average 2.8 hours of television per weekday.[156]

As with overweight and obesity, individuals tend to overestimate their real levels of physical activity, and underestimate their health risks from inactivity. In 2008, only 39 per cent of men and 29 per cent of women reported meeting this minimum level of activity – overweight or obese men and women were less likely to meet these recommendations.[156] In an objective study monitoring activity from wearing an accelerometer, researchers found that only six per cent of men and four per cent of women actually achieved the recommended level of weekly activity. Some insight into this disparity in results might be gleaned from a DH survey, which found that 80 per cent of respondents considered themselves to be 'fairly active' or more, despite the majority not attaining minimum levels of physical activity.[159]

Even among those who had not engaged in any physical activity within the past month, half perceived themselves to be 'fit'.[159]

Summary
Physical inactivity as part of a sedentary lifestyle is a risk factor for cardiovascular disease and obesity, independent of a lack of physical exercise. Although the health benefits of exercise are widely recognised by the public, awareness of the risks of inactivity are less well known. Physical activity levels are low in the UK, and many people overestimate their real activity levels.

Further BMA resources:
- *Transport and health.* British Medical Association (2009).[160]
- *Promoting safe cycling.* British Medical Association (2008).
- *Preventing childhood obesity.* British Medical Association (2005).[154]

3.2.7.   Food and diet
Food has a powerful influence on health. Poor nutritional status is a major contributor to the global burden of disease, from undernourishment, malnutrition and nutritional deficiencies, to energy-dense diets.[111]

The greatest health risk in relation to food is the composition of energy-dense diets rich in saturated fat, sugar and salt.[111] This type of diet is a significant risk factor for many health conditions such as cardiovascular disease, type 2 diabetes, cancer, overweight and obesity.[150, 153] Dietary patterns and food composition have changed significantly in the UK over the past 50 years. The average diet in the UK is now low in fruit and vegetable intake, high in fat and saturated fat intake, sugar and salt intake.[131, 156] The link between food and diet in relation to lifestyle risk factors and diseases such as cardiovascular disease, cancer and diabetes is discussed in detail in sections 3.3.2-3.3.5.

Agricultural and manufacturing processes impact on the composition of diets, and introduce new chemicals into foods. These chemicals include fertilizers, pesticides, preservatives and flavour enhancers. While there is evidence that these chemicals have the potential to cause harm, they can reduce the risk of other harms through the prevention of food contamination and spoilage, and increased food security.[3]

In some countries outside Europe, growth hormones are used in animal husbandry, in particular cattle used for beef or milk production. Hormones accelerate the rate of growth of the animal, or the rate of milk production, and maximise the economic value of the cattle. Six growth hormones are approved by the FDA – estradiol, progesterone, testosterone, zeranol, trenbolone acetate, and melengestrol acetate – as well as one hormone that stimulates milk production. Zeranol, trenoblone acetate and melengestrol acetate are synthetic hormones; whereas the others are naturally-occurring in cattle and humans.[161]

There is concern that residual levels of hormones in meat and milk for human consumption may pose a risk to human health – particularly in young girls and menopausal women, who are particularly sensitive to hormone levels at these stages of life. Following two extensive scientific reviews published in 1999 and 2000, the EC Scientific Committee on Veterinary Measures relating to Public Health (SCVPH) concluded that there may be an association between the use of hormones and increased cancer incidence, and mutagenic effects on human DNA.[162-163] The SCVPH found that information on the effects of hormones in food products is scarce and incomplete, and could not make a clear assessment about health risks or recommend safe levels of hormones in food. In 1999 the committee recommended banning the use of hormones in food production, and a ban on importation of their food products into the EU was introduced.[161-163]

Food contamination is a source of risk to health, from microbial (such as *Salmonella* species (spp), *Escherichia coli*) and chemical (such as dioxins) contaminants. Food contamination can result from poor hygiene, improper handling, inadequate heat treatment and cross contamination from other sources. The increase in pre-prepared food consumption, eating out and international travel are common sources of infection.[164] The most common cause of foodborne outbreaks is from Salmonella, but outbreaks have been in decline since the 1990s, mainly due to improved hygiene practices and food production standards (see **Figure 18**).

The shift towards high-production intensive farming in the 20th century has increased the risk of contamination and ill-health, as evident from the BSE crisis in the 20th century (see page 14).

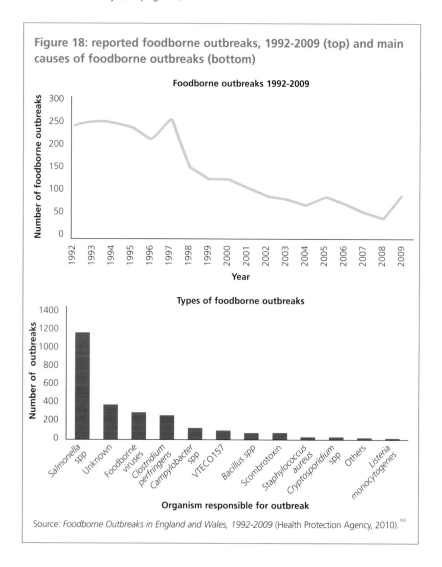

Figure 18: reported foodborne outbreaks, 1992-2009 (top) and main causes of foodborne outbreaks (bottom)

Source: *Foodborne Outbreaks in England and Wales, 1992-2009* (Health Protection Agency, 2010).[165]

Summary

Food scares relating to contamination and new agricultural technologies and practices have led to anxiety about the health risk associated with food. Where the risk to health is not well characterised, the precautionary principle has been adopted in some cases (eg restricting the use and importation of Genetically modified (GM) food and hormones in beef in the EU). In the UK, poor diet is perhaps the greatest risk to health associated with food, in the form of an energy-dense diet, high in sugar, fat and salt.

Further BMA resources:
- *Early life nutrition and lifelong health.* British Medical Association (2009).[155]
- *Preventing childhood obesity.* British Medical Association (2005).[154]
- *Genetically modified foods and health: a second interim statement.* British Medical Association (2004).[166]

3.2.8.   Fertility, pregnancy and childhood

Over the past two centuries, risks in pregnancy, childbirth and infancy have decreased dramatically. For potential harms that affect fertility, pregnancy or infants, there is a tendency to accept lower levels of risk.

Pregnancy, and in particular childbirth, represents a potential health risk to women. The fifth Millenium Development Goal aims to reduce mortality in pregnancy and childbirth by three-quarters by 2015.[167] Between 1990 and 2008, maternal deaths declined 34 per cent globally.[85]

Maternal mortality in the UK is low, at 8.1 deaths per 100,000 live births.[85] Unlike the majority of countries (high and low income), maternal mortality has not decreased over the past 20 years in the UK.[85] A number of health complications commonly occur during pregnancy and childbirth, including ectopic pregnancy, pre-eclampsia and gestational diabetes. The maternal risk factors for these conditions include high blood pressure, obesity, age over 35, and STIs.

There is a long list of foods, chemicals and medicines that pregnant women are urged to avoid, many of which will only minimally reduce the risk of harm to the fetus, but collectively avoidance is likely to result in a healthier pregnancy.

Other more common risks in pregnancy are often not perceived to be as harmful to the fetus as they in fact are. These include smoking, alcohol, obesity and STIs (see **Box 8**).

New mothers may experience postnatal depression, which affects between 10 to 15 women in every 100 births.[168] Onset of postnatal depression commonly occurs in the first six months after childbirth. Like much other depression, postnatal depression is thought to be triggered by major life changes such as the arrival of a new child, new financial constraints and changes to relationships, as well as difficulty or trauma during childbirth.[168]

Prenatal or environmental exposure to estrogenic or anti-androgenic chemicals such as phthalates, bisphenol A (BPA), polychlorinates and dichlorodiphenyltrichloroethane (DDT), among others, has been linked to lower male fertility and endocrine disruption.[169] The use of many of these types of chemicals is being minimised, often as a result of consumer pressure rather than evidence-based public health initiatives. As a precautionary measure, bisphenol A was banned from use in plastic baby bottles in the EU in 2010.[170]

Box 8 – health risks in early life: the BMA perspective

The BMA Board of Science has long recognised the importance of health in early life, from fertility and pregnancy and throughout childhood. The following provides an overview of key messages from Board of Science publications on the health risks in early life.

Fetal alcohol spectrum disorders

The harms of chronic heavy drinking throughout pregnancy have been well-documented. Prenatal alcohol exposure can affect fetal brain and central nervous system development, and lead to intellectual disabilities, physical and emotional development problems, memory and attention disorders, and other behavioural problems. Existing evidence on the harm at low levels of, or occasional, alcohol consumption is inconclusive and there is currently no consensus on the level of risk to the fetus.[171] Given this ambiguity, in its 2007 Board of Science report *Fetal alcohol spectrum disorders – a guide for healthcare professionals* (2007),[139] the BMA recommends that women who are pregnant,

---

or who are considering a pregnancy, should be advised not to consume any alcohol. This recommendation is deliberately conservative due to the precautionary principle – uncertainty as to the outcome of low or moderate drinking in infants.

Early life nutrition and lifelong health

In the 2009 report *Early life nutrition and lifelong health*,[155] the BMA Board of Science recognised the importance of a healthy diet beginning in early life – during pregnancy and infancy – and the impact of early life nutrition on health into adulthood.

Malnutrition not only comprises undernutrition but also inadequate or unbalanced diets. Even in affluent countries such as the UK, many people – including pregnant women – consume poor quality diets that lead to nutritional deficiencies and overweight or obesity. Poor maternal nutrition during pregnancy, and maternal overweight or obesity, are considerable health risks to the child. The lack of breastfeeding during infancy can also lead to obesity, cardiovascular disease, diabetes and other chronic diseases in adulthood. Undernutrition in infancy increases the risk of cognitive disorders and limits physical growth in child- and adulthood. The report noted the importance and value of education and awareness in changing dietary behaviours, such as limiting alcohol consumption, improving nutrition and maintaining a healthy body weight.

Childhood obesity

In 2005, the Board of Science produced its report *Preventing childhood obesity*[154] to highlight the growing health risk of childhood obesity and identify preventive action. It recommended a number of measures, including that:
- the provision of education to parents and children on the elements of healthy living such as balanced diet and physical activity should be improved
- food provided to children in schools should conform to healthy nutritional guidelines
- food manufacturers should be legally obliged to reduce salt, sugar and saturated fat in food products
- access to, and investment in, sports and recreation facilities in schools and communities should be increased.

Smoking and reproductive health

As well as the health risks outlined in previous sections, tobacco smoking also has significant impact on fertility and pregnancy. These health risks were reviewed in the BMA Board of Science report *Smoking and reproductive life* (2004), and include:

- infertility
- reduced response to artificial reproductive treatment
- sperm damage and reduced semen quality
- risk of miscarriage
- risk of ectopic pregnancy
- reduced fetal growth and low birth weight
- premature birth.

In many ways children and infants are more vulnerable to the harms of tobacco smoke than adults: their smaller body weight means they breathe in proportionally more smoke per breath, their lungs and organs are still developing, and their immune system is immature and less capable of defending against toxins in tobacco smoke. Passive smoking is a cause of lower respiratory tract infection, asthma and respiratory problems, middle ear disease, bacterial meningitis and SIDS in children in the UK. The BMA further highlighted these child health risks in its 2007 Board of Science report *Breaking the cycle of children's exposure to tobacco smoke.*[124]

Risks in infancy and childhood

Infancy is recognised as a particularly sensitive period in which parenting and environmental factors can significantly influence a child's future risk of ill health. As noted in **Box 8**, behaviour and practice such as breastfeeding and diet, social and cognitive development, exposure to second hand smoke, air pollution or other toxins, have all been shown to influence health in adulthood. Low birth weight, which is associated with maternal health – including stress, diet, drug, alcohol and tobacco use during pregnancy – can have long-term health and cognitive consequences. A social gradient exists for maternal health status in the UK, where women in the lowest socioeconomic groups have the poorest maternal health. Risk of infant mortality also rises with increasing social deprivation.[122]

Infants under the age of one are at greater risk of death than young children, adolescents and adults.[172] The common underlying causes of death in infants include congenital abnormalities and immaturity-related conditions, infection, asphyxia, anoxia or trauma, SIDS, and other unexplained causes (see **Figure 19**).[173] Less-advantaged infants, toddlers and children are more vulnerable to domestic abuse and neglect, and 17 times more likely to die from accidental or violent causes than those born to parents in professional jobs.[174] Young children are also more vulnerable to a number of risks, in particular accidents such as falls, burns, poisoning, drowning, and road traffic injuries.[3]

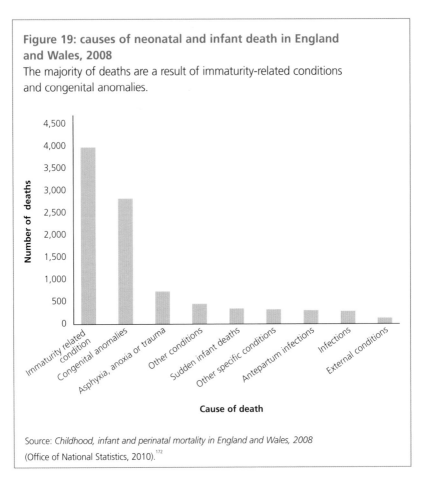

Figure 19: causes of neonatal and infant death in England and Wales, 2008

The majority of deaths are a result of immaturity-related conditions and congenital anomalies.

Source: *Childhood, infant and perinatal mortality in England and Wales, 2008*
(Office of National Statistics, 2010).[172]

Summary

Women and children face a number of unique health risks during pregnancy, childbirth and infancy. Maternal and infant mortality, which are used as indicators of poverty and health inequality, have been reduced in the past century in the UK and worldwide. Where specific risk factors are identified – such as sleeping position of infants and the risk of SIDS – public health campaigns have been successful in reducing infant mortality risk.

Further BMA resources:
- *Early life nutrition and lifelong health.* British Medical Association (2009).[155]
- *Breaking the cycle of children's exposure to tobacco smoke.* British Medical Association (2007).[124]
- *Fetal alcohol spectrum disorders.* British Medical Association (2007).[139]
- *Preventing childhood obesity.* British Medical Association (2005).[154]
- *Growing up in Britain: ensuring a healthy future for our children.* British Medical Association (1999).[175]

3.2.9.   Sports and hobbies

Individuals tend to be willing to accept higher levels of risk when these risks are within their personal control, such as sports and hobbies. Recreational risks can be integral to enjoyment, for example in sport and outdoor activities. High risk sports include contact and ball sports (eg football, rugby, cricket and basketball), water sports (eg boating, canoeing, diving, sailing and swimming) and other sports such as mountaineering, climbing, skiing, snowboarding, and horse riding. Lower risk sports and hobbies include aerobics, athletics, badminton, hiking and dance.[176-177] The most common types of injuries from sports and hobbies include sprains and strains, fractures and dislocations, commonly caused by overextension or strenuous movements.[177-178]

One sport which carries a substantial risk of harm is boxing, which can cause brain damage, haemorrhage, permanent sight or hearing loss, and death.[179] In contrast to the sports mentioned in the preceding paragraph, boxing has the sole aim of causing physical harm to an opponent until they are unable to continue fighting, and professional boxing matches may end in an opponent being knocked unconscious. For this reason, the BMA has campaigned for a ban on boxing since the 1980s, including in its 1993 report, *The Boxing Debate*.

Summary
Risk can be a part of the enjoyment of many sports. The majority of sports are relatively low risk if engaged in properly and with appropriate safety precautions. An important exception is boxing, where the main aim is to cause harm to the opponent and poses significant risks to health.

Further BMA resources:
- *Doctors providing medical care at sporting events.* British Medical Association (2011).[180]
- *Boxing.* British Medical Association (2008).[179]
- *Injury prevention.* British Medical Association (2001).[181]
- *The boxing debate.* British Medical Association (1993).[182]

3.2.10. Accidents and injuries

Injury is a relatively uncommon cause of death in Europe and the UK, and highest among adolescents and young adults, as well as in older people, compared to the general population.[3] There are known risk factors, hazards and predictable patterns of 'accidents'. Common sources of injuries include the home, fire, poisoning, recreational and sports activities, road traffic injuries (see section 3.2.16), suicide, homicide, and violent crime and domestic violence (see section 3.2.12). For many types of accidents and injuries, a social gradient exists where the most socially deprived are at the greatest risk of experiencing an injury.[122]

Fire is a common cause of injury, burns and acute respiratory illness, though an uncommon event in general. Fire incidents and death from fire have been declining over the past 60 years. In 2009, there were nearly 385,000 fires in the UK, of which 52,700 (14%) were in homes and which caused a total of 13,200 casualties. Three quarters of deaths from fires occurred in the home, amounting to 331 deaths.[183] The main sources of fires in the home are cooking appliances, which account for 55 per cent of all fires, and careless handling of fire, for example cigarette disposal, which accounts for 43 per cent of all fires in the home. Consuming alcohol in the home also increases the risk of a serious house fire.[184]

Summary
Risk of death from injury in the UK is low, although minor accidents and injuries are more common. Many injuries occur in the home, including fire-related injuries and deaths.

Further BMA resources:
- *Injury prevention.* British Medical Association (2001).[181]

3.2.11. Violence

Violence, with the intent to cause harm, is an important health risk in young people, in particular young men. The BMA Board of Science reviewed in detail the health risks from, and risk factors for, violence in its 2010 web resource *Violence and health*.

Violence can cause a range of harms to health – from death, injury, disability or chronic pain, to emotional disorders, mental illness and post-traumatic stress disorder.[185] Rape and intimate partner violence can cause complications in pregnancy, miscarriage, low birth rate, premature birth, fetal injury or death, gynaecological disorders, infertility, and STIs, among other harms. Victims of violence are also more likely to engage in risky health behaviours such as alcohol and drug misuse, unsafe sex and smoking.

The risk of being a victim of violence
Violence can include physical violence, domestic abuse and self-harm. In 2009, there were more than two million reported violent incidents in England and Wales.[186] These included nearly 34,000 incidents involving knives and 8,000 incidents involving firearms – a small proportion of all violent incidents.[186]

The average risk across all age groups of being a victim of violence is low. In England, the risk of being a victim of violent crime in 2009/10 was three per cent, however, men were almost twice as likely to have experienced violence (4.2%) than women (1.8%).[186] Young people were at the greatest risk of violence, where the risk in men aged 16 to 24 was 13.3 per cent, and the risk in women of the same age is 4.3 per cent.[186]

Women are more than twice as likely to be victims of domestic violence (0.4%) as men (0.2%).[186] A quarter of women have experienced some form of intimate partner violence or sexual violence in the course of their adult life.[186] Intimate partner violence is common during pregnancy, and half of all cases involve alcohol use.[185] Nearly five per cent of women report having been raped in their adult life, 0.5 per cent in the past year. According to the British Crime Survey this amounts to more than 750,000 victims of rape living in the UK.[186] The vast majority of perpetrators of rape (92%) were known to the victims. The 2007 BMA Board of Science report *Domestic abuse* discusses the physical, psychological, sexual and financial abuse that is common to domestic abuse, as well as the groups most vulnerable to domestic abuse, and the impact it can have on victims and other family members.

Children are also at risk of violence and abuse. The Children Act 1989 defines abuse as causing a child to suffer significant harm to their health or development as a result of the actions of another person.[187] Abuse includes hitting or shaking a child, severe punishment, constant threatening or rejection of a child, sexual assault and neglecting to look after a child.[187] The National Society for the Prevention of Cruelty to Children (NSPCC) estimate that 46,705 children are currently on child protection registers in the UK and at risk of child abuse.[188]

In a survey of 18-24 year olds (young adults) and 11-17 year olds (children), the NSPCC report that 25 per cent of young adults and twenty per cent of children have or had been severely maltreated during their childhood, including severe physical violence, sexual abuse or neglect.[189]

There were 615 homicides and 588 attempted homicides in 2009.[186] The number of suicides is typically one order of magnitude greater (ten times): there were 5,675 suicides reported in 2009 (see **Figure 20**). Self-directed violence, including suicide and self-harm, is an important health risk in young people: suicide is the most common cause of death in young men in the UK.[110] The suicide rate in the UK is 16.8 per 100,000 men and five per 100,000 women. The rate of self harm is 400 per 100,000 population.[110]

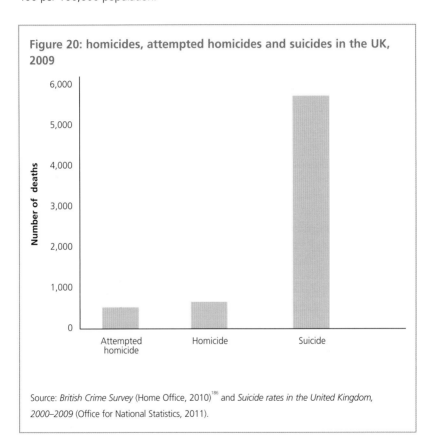

Figure 20: homicides, attempted homicides and suicides in the UK, 2009

Source: *British Crime Survey* (Home Office, 2010)[186] and *Suicide rates in the United Kingdom, 2000–2009* (Office for National Statistics, 2011).

Risk factors for violence perpetration

Young men are more likely to engage in violence: 71 per cent of firearm-related violence, and 72 per cent of alcohol-related violence are perpetrated by young men.[186] Other risk factors for violence perpetration are: a previous experience of violence or abuse, social isolation, unemployment, behavioural disorders, and living in an area of high population density or social inequality.[190]

Alcohol and drug misuse are strongly associated with violence – victims of violence believed that the offender was under the influence of alcohol in 50 per cent of all incidents, and under the influence of drugs in 20 per cent of incidents in 2009.[186]

War and collective violence

Violence includes collective violence such as war, terrorism and state-perpetrated violence including genocide and torture. The WHO definition of collective violence states that it is:

> "the instrumental use of violence by people who identify themselves as members of a group – whether this group is transitory or has a more permanent identity – against another group or set of individuals, in order to achieve political, economic or social objectives."[185]

The 2010 BMA Board of Science web resource *Violence and health* highlights that in the 20th century, 190 million people were killed as a result of collective violence in the 25 largest conflicts. Approximately 60 per cent of these deaths were in the civilian population, many attributable to conflict-related famine and genocide. Collective violence can lead to the displacement of communities and migration of refugees from areas of conflicts.

The WHO estimate that at present, rates of death from collective violence range from less than one in 100,000 per year in some high income countries such as the UK, to 32 per 100,000 per year in Africa.[185] Between 2010-2011, overall mortality rates in the whole of the UK Armed Forces ranged from 71 to 107 per 100,000 personnel, with up to 134 deaths per 100,000 in the Army.[191]

There are a number of known risk factors for collective violence, which can interact to create conditions that lead to violence. These can include:

- inequality
- lack of democratic process
- political instability
- severe economic decline
- deterioration of public services
- rapidly changing population demographics, such as increasing population density or youth
- ethnic composition of the ruling group being different to that of the general population
- cycles of violent revenge
- availability of small arms.[185]

There are a number of other health consequences of collective violence, beyond mortality and morbidity of those involved in conflicts. These can include increased infant mortality, the spread of communicable diseases, mental health disorders in the population, poverty, increased refugees and displaced populations, and significant impacts on the provision of, and access to healthcare services and infrastructure.[185]

Summary

Young people are at greatest risk of being a victim of violence, especially young men. Relative to homicide, the risk of death from suicide is under-recognised in the UK. Women are more than twice as likely to be victims of domestic violence as men.

Further BMA resources:
- *Violence and health*. British Medical Association (2010).[190]
- *Domestic abuse*. British Medical Association (2007).[192]

3.2.12.   Occupational risk

Employment can be a source of health risks, and is dependent on the nature of tasks involved.

Occupational risks

Occupational hazards can include exposure to chemicals, the working environment, machinery and transport vehicles, and hazards associated with specific industries. These can lead to injury and death as well as chronic conditions such as COPD or cancer. High risk industries include agriculture, construction, transport, fisheries, energy, chemicals and manufacturing. Within these industries skilled labourers and machine operators are at greatest risk of injury.

Many of the occupational health effects observed are a result of exposure to chemicals and carcinogens in the past, when working conditions were less safe. In younger workers who have experienced better working conditions throughout their employment, prevalence of work-related illness is significantly lower.[193]

As a result of greater exposure to a range of hazards, the most significant occupational health risks in the UK are to those working in the energy industry, from accidents and injury to chronic health conditions. While safety has improved, coal mining and off-shore drilling remain, in relative terms, highly dangerous occupations.

Nuclear energy has other significant occupational and public health risks. Mining uranium, the raw material of nuclear energy, carries similar health risks to coal and other mining in miners. Occupational exposure to ionising radiation is also associated with a small increase in cancers, in particular prostate cancer.[194] Commercial pilots and airline staff are exposed to higher levels of cosmic radiation, however it is estimated that their increased risk of cancer from cosmic radiation over a lifetime is negligible (see section 3.5.3).[195]

In 2008, there were 180 deaths at work from injury, an incidence rate of 0.6 per 100,000 workers in Great Britain.[193] There were between 132,000 and 246,000 reported injuries to employees.[193] It is estimated that approximately 8,000 cancer deaths per year can be attributed to occupation exposure to carcinogens in Great Britain.[196] Approximately 4,000 of these cancer deaths are attributed to past exposure to asbestos, of which more than 2,100 were from mesothelioma in 2007.[196]

The most common occupational risks are musculoskeletal disorders and mental disorders.[193, 197] Approximately 400,000 workers suffer from work-related stress including anxiety or depression.[193] Stress at work is itself a risk factor for other health conditions such as alcohol dependence, obesity and CHD. Despite these consequences, stress at work is not widely recognised as an important occupational health risk by employees and employers alike.

Occupational health risks may also include working unsocial hours and shift working, which doctors are often required to do when providing out-of-hours care, emergency care, when on call or during their training. The BMA report *Health effects of working unsocial hours and shift work*[198] highlights the negative health consequences of variable and unsocial shift patterns, which include a disruption to sleep patterns and circadian rhythms, and altered eating patterns.[199] Circadian rhythm disruption can impact on physiological processes such as respiratory, cardiovascular, digestive and renal function, as well as body temperature, hormone production, the menstrual cycle and cell division. Changes in eating behaviour and a disruption of meal times can lead to increased body mass index (BMI) and risk of obesity in shift workers.[198]

Employment as a protective factor
Good quality employment[e] is also very good for health, and can be considered a protective factor, meeting many of an individual's mental health needs as well as economic ones. These include many psychosocial needs such as full participation in society, reward, satisfaction, control, identity and social status.

---

e Good quality employment demonstrates that the workforce is valued, protecting against adverse working conditions and enabling a good work-life balance. Practical ways of achieving good quality employment involve complying with UK employment and safety legislation, in particular the Health and Safety at Work etc Act 1974, the Management of Health and Safety at Work Regulations 1999, and the Workplace (Health, Safety and Welfare) Regulations 1992. Briefly, employers have a duty to make the workplace safe and comfortable, and prevent risks to health. Measures to minimise health risks include the safe use of machinery and materials, the provision of first aid facilities, adequate training and supervision to handle hazardous materials and manage hazardous situations, suitable ventilation, temperature, cleanliness, lighting, toilet and rest facilities. Good working conditions also encompass basic employment rights such as minimum wage, working hour limits, entitlements to annual leave, sickness leave, and maternity or paternity leave.

People in work are in better health.[200] Socioeconomic health inequality is related to many factors including employment.[201] Employment status is a key driver of the social determinants of health, and is linked to mental health and mortality. Dame Carol Black's 2008 report *Working for a healthier tomorrow* identified that individuals who are unemployed have poorer general health, higher consumption of medication, and more healthcare visits than those in employment (even after accounting for those who are unable to work due to chronic limiting medical condition).[202] Employment can influence an individual's social position, and lead to greater psychological wellbeing, and reduced mental health disorders such as depression and anxiety.[202-203]

Employment can raise an individual's socioeconomic status and is a key source of income, which is also linked to health. The Marmot review highlighted that an income gradient exists where lower incomes can lead to poorer health.[122] Those on lower incomes purchase cheaper goods and services that may have increased health risks, and are less able to purchase goods and services that improve health.[122] Individuals with low incomes lose on average 17 years of disability-free life, compared to individuals with high incomes, due to worse living conditions. Poor health can also reduce employment opportunities and earning potential.[122] Children of parents on low income or who are unemployed also have poorer health and educational outcomes, compared to children of parents on higher incomes.[122]

Summary

In general, good quality employment is a protective factor for health. Musculoskeletal disorders and stress are the most common occupational-related illnesses. Many occupational hazards exist, especially in certain industries such as energy, manufacturing and construction. Employers have a responsibility to minimise the risk of injury and ill-health in the workplace. Psychological hazards of work, especially low levels of work autonomy, seem to have a substantial role in overall health.

3.2.13. Housing and air pollution

Housing can be the source of many hazards, exposure to which is exacerbated by the large proportion of time spent in them. These can range from the materials, chemicals, appliances and structure of houses, and can have a broad range of health consequences, from falls, burns, and poisoning to chronic ill health.

As highlighted in the BMA Board of Science report *Housing and Health: building for the future* (2003), poor housing quality, overcrowding and unsanitary conditions can increase the risk of the spread of communicable diseases and exacerbate indoor air pollution. These conditions are risk factors for general ill health and are frequently associated with poverty.

Poorly heated homes and fuel poverty are risks to health. A household is living in fuel poverty when it needs to spend more than ten per cent of its income on the cost of fuel. Fuel poverty and cold homes were associated with 25,400 excess winter deaths in the UK in 2009/10, as well as increased cardiovascular and respiratory illnesses, colds and flu, and mental disorders.[204] Fuel poverty also restricts dietary opportunities and choices due to competing financial pressures on a limited income.[204]

Indoor air quality can have an important impact on health – unsurprisingly as Europeans spend as much as 90 per cent of their time indoors. A range of airborne chemicals such as volatile inorganic compounds (VOCs), nitrogen dioxide, particulate matter, and carbon monoxide are associated with adverse health effect such as cancer, allergy and asthma and skin irritation.[205] Asbestos and other building materials have also been linked to cancer and ill health. An important source of air pollution in the UK is radon gas (see section 3.5.3), which enters buildings from the ground beneath. Adequate ventilation is necessary to keep concentrations of VOCs and other gases low in the home.

In the developing world, indoor air quality and inhalation of smoke from solid fuels (coal, charcoal, dung, wood or crop residues) is a major source of respiratory disease and infection. It accounts for almost three per cent of the burden of disease in low income countries, but has a negligible effect on health in high income countries.[112-113]

The main source of outdoor air pollution is road transport, specifically vehicle emission of pollutants including nitrogen oxides, VOCs, carbon monoxide, sulphur dioxide, ground level ozone and particulate matter. Outdoor air pollution increases the risk of respiratory diseases including asthma, cardiovascular disease and ischaemic heart disease, as well as premature death.[206-209] Air pollution from transport has also been shown to increase the risk of premature birth and negatively affect child development.[206]

Summary
Poor housing quality is a risk factor for general ill health and the spread of infectious disease. Household fuel poverty increases the risk of illness and excess winter deaths. Outdoor air pollution, primarily from road transport, increases the risk of respiratory and cardiovascular illnesses, as well as premature death.

Further BMA resources:
- *Transport and health.* British Medical Association (2009).[160]
- *Housing and health: building for the future.* British Medical Association (2003).[210]

3.2.14. Mobile phones
Since they became widespread in their use, there has been concern over the effects of microwave radiation from mobile phones and mobile phone masts, and in particular whether there is a risk of causing diseases such as brain cancer. This did not prevent the use of mobile phones being widely adopted, almost universally across the globe, due to their significant benefits to communication and inexpensive cost.

There is insufficient evidence to suggest that the vast uptake of mobile phone use has resulted in a concomitant increase in brain cancers. The WHO 2010 Interphone Study – which gathered international evidence on mobile phone use over a ten year period – did not find any evidence that mobile phone use increases the risk of brain tumours.[211] As mobile phones have only been in common use for a little more than a decade, the study was not able to draw any conclusions on the long-term health risk.[211] A recent study of more than 350,000 Danish men and women similarly found no association with mobile phone use and increased incidence of cancers of the nervous system.[212]

The Interphone Study confirmed the findings of a 2000 review by the UK Independent Expert Group on Mobile Phones, which concluded that there was little evidence of adverse health outcomes from mobile phone usage or phone masts.[211] The review found that public exposure to radiofrequency (RF) radiation from mobile phones and phone masts was below recommended guidelines and would not be expected to cause adverse health effects in the general population. The Group did not, however, rule out the possibility that certain individuals could be more sensitive to RF exposure and predisposed to ill-health, and recommended a precautionary approach until this possibility could be ruled out. The review also concluded that mobile phone use while driving posed a significant risk of road traffic crashes.

The BMA Board of Science report *Mobile phones* (2001) similarly recommended a precautionary approach to mobile phones, while recognising that no major adverse health effects associated with mobile phone use or mobile phone masts had yet been reported.

Summary
Mobile phones are unlikely to pose a significant risk to health. The widespread benefits of mobile phone use in terms of communication outweigh the risk of harm.

Further BMA resources:
- *Mobile phones and health: an interim report.* British Medical Association (2001).[213]

3.2.15.   Infectious diseases and pandemic influenza

Infectious diseases – such as lower respiratory tract infection, diarrhoeal diseases, HIV, malaria and tuberculosis – remain the leading causes of death in low income countries, whereas in middle and high income countries they have been superseded by the non-communicable diseases.

Zoonotic diseases (those that are transmissible from animal to human) include bacteria (eg *E. coli*), parasites (eg cysticercosis/taeniasis, or tapeworm), fungi (eg dermatophytoses, or ringworm), viruses (eg Rabies) and prions (eg BSE prions). Infectious diseases can also be transmitted via bites from insects carrying diseases such as mosquitoes (malaria, dengue fever, West Nile virus, yellow fever), fleas (plague) and ticks (Lyme disease).

Infectious disease in the UK

The prevalence of infectious disease in the UK is low relative to low and middle income countries, and infectious diseases account for approximately one per cent of deaths per year in England and Wales.[110] The prevalence of certain infections can be higher among certain demographic groups, such as migrants, although even in these groups overall prevalence is generally low.[214] In 2004, for example, 70 per cent of tuberculosis and HIV cases reported in England and 70 per cent of malaria cases in the UK were acquired outside of the UK, but the prevalence of tuberculosis in non-UK born population remained low, at 94 per 100,000 population.[214] Many infections are likely acquired prior to arrival in the UK, and the HPA estimate that the risk of significant levels of transmission to the wider UK population of infectious diseases acquired prior to arrival in the UK is low.[214]

The prevalence and infection rate of infectious diseases can be higher in closed communities such as prisons.[215-216] Prevalence of tuberculosis, HIV, hepatitis B and C and sexually transmitted infections are higher in prisons than in the general population.[216-217] Transmission of infectious diseases within prisons is higher due to risk factors such as injecting drug use, unsafe sex, unsafe practices such as tattooing, overcrowding and poor ventilation.[216] In the UK, prisoners with tuberculosis were more likely to have a drug-resistant strain than individuals with tuberculosis in the general population.[215]

Seasonal influenza

The influenza viruses are responsible for common seasonal flu. They also have the potential to cause a global pandemic as they are capable of rapid mutation and generation of novel viruses. It is spread easily by airborne, direct and indirect transmission – such as through physical contact, coughing and sneezing.

Seasonal influenza in humans is a subtype of the influenza virus, to which humans have partial immunity through chronic exposure. In this form it is capable of causing illness and premature death – up to 500,000 deaths worldwide each year – in particular in older people and those with underlying health problems.[218] For most periods of the year, most people are at limited risk of infection and illness from the influenza virus. This risk increases during the flu season, but even over this period the risk of serious illness or death remains low for the majority of the population, where mainly young children under four years of age, and adults over 80 years of age are at higher risk (see **Figure 21**).[219]

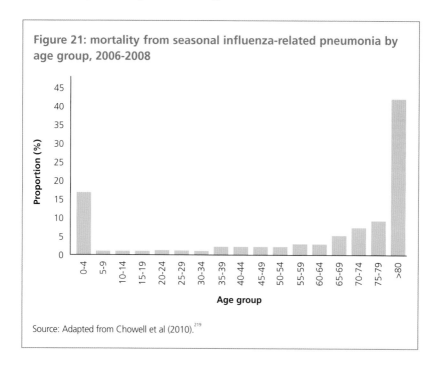

Figure 21: mortality from seasonal influenza-related pneumonia by age group, 2006-2008

Source: Adapted from Chowell et al (2010).[219]

Pandemic influenza

Influenza is a common infection in humans as well as animals including birds (avian) and pigs (swine). It is rare for the virus to mutate and become transmissible to humans from animals. Where animal to human transmission has been documented, the effects are typically severe because humans have little or no prior exposure to the virus and no immune protection. A pandemic can develop rapidly if the novel influenza virus mutates further and becomes transmissible from human to human.

Pandemic influenza is defined by the WHO as a situation where the influenza virus mutates into a new form, is capable of spreading from human to human, and causes serious illness:

> *"An influenza pandemic may occur when a new influenza virus appears against which the human population has no immunity"*[220]

The likelihood that a pandemic will occur increases with every animal to human transmission event, which represent opportunities for the virus to mutate into a form more pathogenic to humans. The risk of infection, illness and death to the individual, remains very low between pandemics.

Pandemic influenza can spread rapidly across borders and around the world. Infection rates can reach 25 to 35 per cent of the population in affected regions.[218, 221] **Table 4** records the major pandemics of the past century. With the current knowledge of influenza it is not possible to predict the severity of illness that a new subtype of influenza will cause. In terms of risk management, pandemic influenza is an example of a risk with a high degree of intrinsic uncertainty; it is by definition an emerging disease (see **Box 9**).

Table 4 – historic pandemics

Pandemic	Area of emergence	Influenza A virus type	Estimated case fatality rate	Estimated attributable excess worldwide mortality (people)	Groups most affected
1918 Spanish Influenza	Unknown	H1N1	2-3%	20-50 million	Young adults
1957-1958 Asian Flu	Southern China	H2N2	<0.2%	1-4 million	Children
1968-1969 Hong Kong Flu	Southern China	H3N2	<0.2%	1-4 million	All age groups
2008-2009 Pandemic (H1N1)	Mexico	H1N1	0.04%	>18,000 (laboratory confirmed cases)	Infants, pregnant women

Avian influenza

The avian influenza virus (bird flu) is common among birds, and can be highly pathogenic in domestic birds. The avian influenza virus does not normally infect humans. It can occur very rarely from direct, close contact with infected poultry, in particular in semi-rural households where free range poultry share living spaces with humans. Avian influenza symptoms in humans can be aggressive and fatal (for example pneumonia, severe respiratory disease and organ failure), with rapid deterioration and high fatality.[222]

While rare transmission of avian influenza from poultry to humans is an important health risk, of far greater risk is the potential of the virus to mutate into a form that is transmissible by person to person contact, initiating a highly virulent pandemic influenza. The more often the virus is transmitted from bird to human, the more opportunity it has to mutate. Avian influenza is now endemic in poultry in Indonesia, Vietnam, Cambodia, China and Thailand, increasing the probability of animal to human transmission and viral mutation into a pandemic form.

Pandemic H1N1 2009

The influenza virus caused the 2009 pandemic. The novel influenza virus subtype of H1N1 may have originated in Mexico in April 2009, and rapidly spread across the world, to more than 200 countries and overseas territories, infecting up to 15 per cent of the population in affected regions.[219, 223-224]

Worldwide, there were more than 18,000 confirmed deaths from the H1N1 2009 pandemic, verified through laboratory tests, which was relatively low compared to historic pandemics. Globally, nearly 30 per cent of deaths were in people with no underlying health conditions, and nearly 80 per cent of deaths occurred in people under 65 years of age, in comparison to seasonal flu in which mortality is concentrated in the over-65s (over 90% of deaths). **Figure 22** illustrates the epidemiological differences between the H1N1 pandemic and seasonal flu.[219, 225]

In the UK, the total number of confirmed deaths from the pandemic influenza was 474. Of these, 35 were in children under five years of age, and 15 in pregnant women.[223] At its peak in November 2009, the estimated incidence rate of influenza in the UK was over 150 people per 100,000 population per week (see **Box 9**).[223]

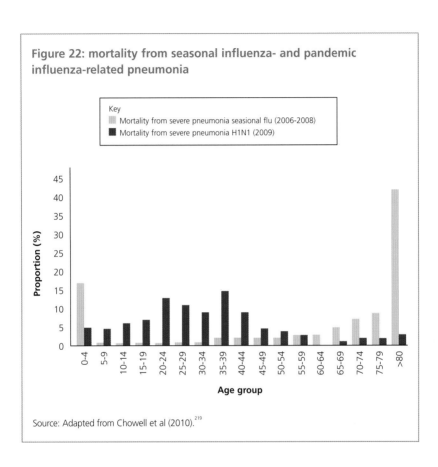

Figure 22: mortality from seasonal influenza- and pandemic influenza-related pneumonia

Key
▨ Mortality from severe pneumonia seasonal flu (2006-2008)
■ Mortality from severe pneumonia H1N1 (2009)

Source: Adapted from Chowell et al (2010).[219]

Box 9 – risk management and pandemic preparedness in the UK

From its emergence in April 2009, to being officially declared over in August 2010, pandemic preparedness risk management strategies were put into action in the UK and globally. The Cabinet Office coordinated the national response in the UK, with input from the devolved administrations' health departments and CMOs, and the HPA. The BMA was active in communication between front line medical staff and the central response, and played a role in providing clear and authoritative clinical advice.

The UK has developed a framework for dealing with health emergencies, both 'big bang' and 'rising tide'. This framework includes the government obtaining the best advice on how to reduce the risks of the most serious consequences of a pandemic, and the use of clear risk assessment, management and mitigation strategies.

While it was inevitable that the pandemic flu virus would reach the UK, strategies to reduce its transmission within the population were put in place. This gave time for the development of knowledge on treatment, viral identification, and supporting progress towards vaccine production.

As part of its pandemic preparedness strategy, the UK had built a stockpile of antiviral drugs. Although there were some concerns over the side effects of the antiviral drug Oseltamivir,[226] initial studies indicated that the benefits of the drug – it was effective in reducing the duration and severity of influenza in patients – outweighed the risk of adverse reactions.[227-228]

The UK also had a pre-existing order for sufficient vaccine stocks to vaccinate the entire population against the influenza virus in the event of a pandemic, as a method of decreasing transmission. Once the virus strain was identified and isolated, a vaccine was rapidly developed. With new epidemiological information on the evolving pandemic influenza, the UK Government took the decision to start by vaccinating those at high risk, including young children and pregnant women. Despite acquiring more vaccines than eventually needed, the vaccines were deemed to be cost effective in relation to lives saved. Subsequent studies demonstrated that the vaccines were safe, with minimal side effects, and the benefits of immunisation outweighed the risks to the individual, particularly in high risk groups.[229]

The effectiveness of the containment strategy of school closures, with the aim of decreasing transmission of the virus, was variable. Research from Hong Kong suggests that school closures reduced transmission of the influenza virus by 25 per cent, but in the UK school closures were resource-intensive and eventually abandoned.[229]

The government invested heavily in risk communication, emphasising risk reduction strategies such as 'catch it, kill it, bin it', and on explanations of their policies on vaccines and antivirals. There were some successes, but there is much to learn from this strategy. Additionally the government targeted preventative measures at first responders and health care workers. Evidence from analysis of severe acute respiratory syndrome (SARS) had shown an excess risk to this groups, leading to a targeted response.

In the post-pandemic period, Dame Deirdre Hine undertook an independent review of the UK Government's implementation of the pandemic preparedness strategy, and concluded that the risk management strategy that had been in place since 2005 had ensured that the UK was well-prepared to manage its response to the pandemic. The review acknowledged the "inherent… unpredictability of the influenza virus" and noted that given this uncertainty, the pandemic response was "proportionate and effective" in terms of economic costs and the wider costs to society.[224]

In the aftermath of the pandemic, concern was expressed that the broad definition of a "pandemic" adopted by the WHO does not adequately take into account its severity, in this case leading to a "false alarm" and a disproportionate public health response by governments worldwide.[230] In response, the WHO disagreed that the pandemic response was an overreation, and reiterated that the virus met the criteria for pandemics: it was a novel virus to which humans showed no immunity, displaced existing strains and it had novel patterns of infection, illness and death in humans. The WHO stated that severity was not included in the criteria for pandemic because it was subject to change over time, across populations and geographic locations.[231]

Summary
Most people, at most times, are at low risk of seasonal influenza, and very low risk of pandemic influenza. During influenza epidemics, some vulnerable groups are at higher risk, including infants and the elderly. For these groups, greater precautions such as encouraging vaccination can reduce the risk of infection.

The likelihood of a future pandemic is almost certain. As demonstrated during the 2009 pandemic, disaster preparedness and the implementation of defined risk management strategies are essential for minimising the risk of infection and illness in the general population. Cooperation and coordination between many organisations, including the health services, are integral to a successful pandemic preparedness plan.

3.2.16. Road transport

Transport, by any mode, is generally a safe activity in the UK. There is substantial variation in transport health risks, dependent on transport mode, as well as inconsistent perceptions of risk. Aviation is the mode of transport with the lowest statistical risk of mortality or injury.

Road transport – by car, motorcycle, bus, walking and cycling – is in general a low-risk activity. It is also extremely common – most people drive, walk or cycle at least a short distance everyday. The risk of injury is extremely low for any given journey, but the cumulative risk of injury over a lifetime of transport is comparatively high: the lifetime risk of being injured in a road traffic crash is between one in two and one in three.[232]

Injury and death are the main health risks associated with road transport, as well as the chronic health effects of air pollution, in particular in middle income countries. As highlighted in the 2009 BMA Board of Science briefing paper *Transport and Health*,[f] the common risk factors for road traffic injury and death are: driving under the influence of alcohol or drugs, speeding, fatigue or distraction. External factors such as road design, environmental conditions and poor weather can also influence the risk of crashes. The type of road influences the risk of a road traffic crash – crashes are more common on urban roads than rural roads or motorways, per billion passenger mile (**Figure 23**).[233]

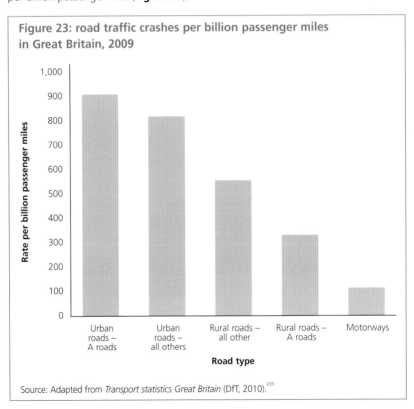

Figure 23: road traffic crashes per billion passenger miles in Great Britain, 2009

Source: Adapted from *Transport statistics Great Britain* (DfT, 2010).[233]

---

f   The BMA Board of Science is currently developing a report that will present up-to-date research and evidence on sustainable transport, with a focus on the future anticipated challenges in sustainable transport and health, and addressing government policy in this area. It is planned that this will be published in mid 2012.

In the UK, mortality and injury from road traffic crashes for all road users has declined sharply in the past 60 years (see **Figure 24**). There were estimated to be 1,800 deaths, 24,510 serious injuries and more than 208,648 injuries in total in Great Britain in 2010. Travel by motorcycle is the highest risk mode of road transport, killing 89 motorcyclists per billion passenger kilometres in 2008, compared to 31 for pedestrians, 24 for cyclists, and three for car drivers.[234]

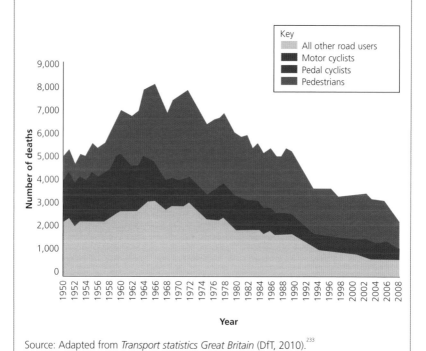

Figure 24: road casualties by mode of transport in Great Britain, 1950-2008

Risk of death from road traffic incidents has declined for all transport modes since its peak in the 1960s.

Source: Adapted from *Transport statistics Great Britain* (DfT, 2010).[233]

Per journey or kilometre, pedestrians and cyclists are more at risk of death or injury than car occupants.[235] As walking and cycling become more common in some cities, the risk of injury per pedestrian or cyclist per mile decreases.[135, 236] This phenomenon is known as the "safety in numbers" effect.

Although there are some road safety risks associated with walking and cycling, there are also substantial benefits to health (predominantly from increased physical activity). In its 1994 report *Cycling towards health and safety*, the BMA calculated that the benefits to health gained from cycling outweigh the risks of injury and death by a factor of 20 to 1. Recent studies found that the health benefits of cycling are greater than the risk of road traffic injuries in the population.[237-238]

Other transport modes
Rail and commercial aviation are exceptionally safe modes of travel, compared to road safety per mile or journey (see **Figure 25**). The average number of fatalities per billion vehicle miles per year is 6.9 for road transport in the UK, 0.2 for rail transport and can be as low as zero for commercial aviation in years where no plane crashes have occurred.[233] These data are complicated by differences in passenger numbers and journey distance, but underline the low risk of rail and commercial aviation.

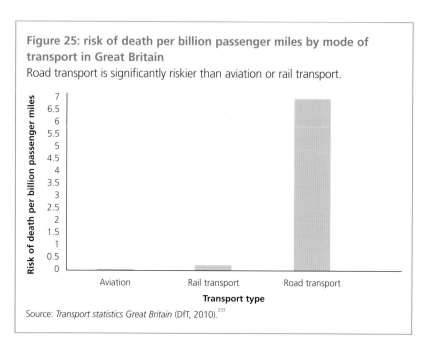

Figure 25: risk of death per billion passenger miles by mode of transport in Great Britain

Road transport is significantly riskier than aviation or rail transport.

Source: *Transport statistics Great Britain* (DfT, 2010).[233]

The low risk of rail and commercial aviation is due to stringent risk management and safety practices that are in place, as well as the controlled environment in which they operate. Rail and aviation casualties occur, and because a single event affects a large number of people at once, and is outside their personal control, the public perception of the risks of rail or aviation can be amplified. This is an example of availability bias: air and rail crashes are readily recalled, leading to the perception that they are more common.

Aviation passengers (and airline staff) are exposed to an increased level of ionising radiation from cosmic radiation at higher altitudes and x-ray scanners used at airport security stations. A recent study estimated the additional health risks of aviation from increased exposure to radiation and concluded that they were negligible relative to normal exposure to natural and medical sources of radiation, and did not significantly increase the risk of developing cancer (see section 3.5.3).[195]

Long haul flights may increase the risk of deep vein thrombosis (DVT) in the lower limbs and pulmonary embolism, which can be fatal. Although the risk of DVT is relatively low, the increase in long haul flights, and the increase in passengers with underlying health conditions will all contribute to DVT becoming a more common risk of flying. These and other risks of flying, including spread of infections, are reviewed in the BMA Board of Science report *The impact of flying on passenger health* (2004). Travel to the airport remains the most risky part of the journey.

Summary
The lifetime risk of injury and death from road transport is relatively high compared to other common activities. Although the UK has a good safety record within the EU, there are still more than 2,000 people killed on British roads every year. Pedestrians and cyclists are vulnerable road users in particular. As a result of the acknowledged benefits of transport in terms of access and mobility, public acceptance of its risks is high. In contrast to road transport, the risk of death or injury from rail and aviation is much lower per passenger mile.

Further BMA resources:
- *Transport and health.* British Medical Association (2009).[160]
- *Driving under the influence of drugs.* British Medical Association (2009).[239]
- *Promoting safe cycling.* British Medical Association (2008).[240]
- *Alcohol misuse: tackling the UK epidemic.* British Medical Association (2008).[126]

3.3. Everyday medical risks

3.3.1. Mental health
Mental health disorders are common in the UK, with an estimated one in four people experiencing a mental health problem each year.[241] Anxiety and depression are the most common disorders. Poor mental health is also a risk factor for self-harm and suicide (see section 3.2.11)

Many of the everyday lifestyle and medical risks described in the previous section, as well as risks in the environment, can affect mental health. Alcohol and drug misuse, physical inactivity, coping with dementia or cancer, or experiencing a natural disaster such as a major flood, storm or earthquake can contribute to the development of mental health disorders.

Physical illness can trigger mental health disorders including depression and anxiety, and post-traumatic stress disorder (PTSD). Physical illness is stressful and can lead to feelings of loss of control, helplessness, isolation and loneliness. In some cases, the drugs used to treat illness can affect brain pathways involved in emotion (eg steroids) and contribute directly to anxiety and depression. Pain from physical illnesses can also contribute to depression and anxiety.[242]

The Royal College of Psychiatrists (RCPsych) highlight that the onset of PTSD can be triggered by diagnosis with a life-threatening illness, being involved in (or witnessing) a serious road accident, exposure to war and conflict, being physically or sexually abused, or from the unexpected injury or death of a close friend or family member.[242] In these instances, approximately one third of those affected go on to develop PTSD.[242]

Financial insecurity and debt are associated with risk of mental disorders. At the individual level, major life events – such as property ownership, marriage, divorce and retirement – can lead to financial insecurity.

A high burden of consumer debt is a known risk factor for mental health disorders including anxiety and depression. The RCPsych conducted a literature review of the relationship between debt and mental health, and found that individuals living in debt are up to four times more likely to experience mental illness: the greater the amount of debt, the greater their risk of mental illnesses compared to those who are not in debt.[242-243] Nearly two out of three people in debt have common mental disorders, and debt can have a wider impact on an individual's sense of identity, social and family relationships. In the current econimic climate, the RCPsych predict that more people will experience financial and job insecurity, and expects that the incidence of mental disorders will increase concurrently in the population.[242]

Financial insecurity and debt are independently associated with depression.[244] Between 35 and 80 per cent of people in mortgage arrears experience depression – in 2009, approximately two per cent of all mortgage holders were in arrears.[243] Data from recent research cited in the Government Office for Science Foresight report *Mental capital and wellbeing* suggest that the established link between low income and mental disorders is largely accounted for by debt rather than income status.[245-246] Existing mental disorders can be exacerbated by job insecurity, debt, poverty, low quality housing and stressful working conditions.[244]

Some groups of people are more likely to experience mental health disorders: approximately 2 in 5 people living in elderly care homes experience depression, and 90 per cent of prisoners have a mental disorder.[242] Approximately 10 per cent of children experience mental health problems.[242]

Summary
Mental health disorders are common in the general population in the UK. Major life events, such as a life-threatening illness, experiencing a natural disaster, and financial pressures, can increase the risk of mental health disorders.

Further BMA resources:
- *The psychological and social needs of inpatients.* British Medical Association (2011).[247]
- *Child and adolescent mental health: a guide for healthcare professionals.* British Medical Association (2006).[248]

3.3.2. High blood pressure (hypertension)
Hypertension is a major risk factor for many cardiovascular diseases including stroke and CHD, and renal disease. It is strongly associated with other diseases and risk factors such as diabetes and obesity, and is a significant health risk in middle and high income countries. The prevalence of hypertension in the UK population is approximately 30 per cent.[131]

High dietary salt intake is one of the main risk factors for hypertension.[249-251] The current recommended daily salt intake in the UK is 6g or less. A 2008 study estimates that 82 per cent of men and 65 per cent of women consume more than 6g per day, with mean daily salt intake at 9.7g for men and 7.7g for women (see **Figure 26**).[252] The main sources of salt in adult diets are in processed foods such as cereal (30%), meat (28%), and dairy products (8%).[252]

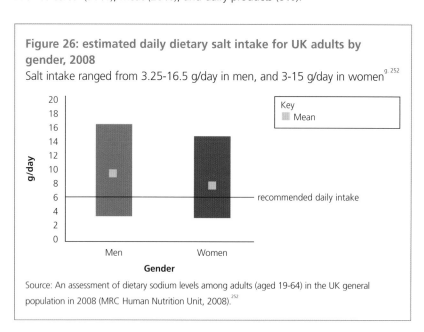

Figure 26: estimated daily dietary salt intake for UK adults by gender, 2008

Salt intake ranged from 3.25-16.5 g/day in men, and 3-15 g/day in women[g. 252]

Source: An assessment of dietary sodium levels among adults (aged 19-64) in the UK general population in 2008 (MRC Human Nutrition Unit, 2008).[252]

A number of studies have suggested that reducing daily salt intake is effective at reducing blood pressure. This association is not restricted to those with hypertension or high salt intake – blood pressure decreases with lower salt intake even in people within the normal blood pressure range (normotensive). Weight reduction, reduction in alcohol intake, increased physical activity and a high fibre diet are other effective measures to reduce blood pressure.[249-251]

Summary

Hypertension is a risk factor for cardiovascular and renal diseases, and is common in the UK population. High dietary salt intake is one of the main risk factors for hypertension.

g   95 per cent of study participants had daily salt intake within these ranges.

3.3.3. Cardiovascular disease

Cardiovascular diseases are the commonest cause of premature death worldwide, and are a major contributor to the global burden of disease. They are a group of disorders that affect the circulatory system (the heart and blood vessels), and include CHD, stroke and other cerebrovascular diseases, myocardial infarction, atherosclerosis, and peripheral vascular disease.

Many of the disorders that comprise cardiovascular disease share the same underlying, and largely preventable, risk factors described previously: high blood pressure, tobacco and alcohol use, high cholesterol, poor diet, overweight, obesity and physical inactivity. [111, 115]

Cardiovascular disease is the cause of over a third of all deaths annually in the UK. Stroke and CHD account for three quarters of all deaths from cardiovascular disease.[110] Although they remain a major cause of mortality, deaths from cardiovascular disease have been in decline in the UK over the past 40 years. One study estimated that approximately 60 per cent of this decline could be attributed to prevention, through the reduction or elimination of risk factors, primarily smoking tobacco. The remaining 40 per cent of the decline was attributed to improved clinical treatment of cardiovascular disease.[253]

A social gradient exists in which cardiovascular disease is increasingly prevalent in lower socioeconomic status individuals, as are many of the cardiovascular disease risk factors – greater waist-hip ratios, lower high density lipoprotein (HDL) cholesterol, lower respiratory fitness, higher diabetes prevalence, and increased likelihood to smoke.[254] Behavioural and psychosocial risk factors in low socioeconomic status individuals, such as low job grade, stress and health behaviours, influence cardiovascular disease risk, as well as parental socioeconomic status, early-life experiences and inequalities in access to health services.[255]

Summary
Cardiovascular disease is the most common cause of premature death, worldwide and in the UK. There are a number of known preventable risk factors for cardiovascular disease, including tobacco and alcohol use, hypertension, overweight and obesity, physical inactivity, and poor diet.

3.3.4.   Cancer risk

Cancer Research UK estimates that the lifetime risk of developing cancer is one in three. In the UK, cancer is the cause of approximately one quarter of all deaths annually, more than 156,000 in 2008.[256] This equates to an annual death rate of 208 people per 100,000 population in the UK. There is a wide variation across the different types of cancer, the different rates of cancer prevalence across age groups, and variation according to the known lifestyle risk factors such as diet, tobacco use, obesity, and unsafe sex.

The risk of cancer diagnosis or death is much higher in older age groups. In 2008, over 300,000 new cases of cancer were diagnosed in the UK. Of these, more than a third (36%) were diagnosed in people aged 75 and over; and more than three out of five in those aged 65 and over (see **Figure 27**).[256] A similar trend is seen with cancer mortality, which is concentrated in older age groups. This partly reflects the cumulative damage to cells that occurs over a lifetime, which can trigger cancer. Cancer and cancer mortality is therefore much rarer in those aged under 60, and only one per cent of cancer diagnoses are in children under 14 years old.[256]

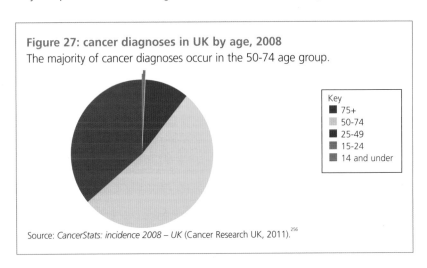

Figure 27: cancer diagnoses in UK by age, 2008
The majority of cancer diagnoses occur in the 50-74 age group.

Key
- ■ 75+
- ▨ 50-74
- ■ 25-49
- ■ 15-24
- ■ 14 and under

Source: *CancerStats: incidence 2008 – UK* (Cancer Research UK, 2011).[256]

Cancer is a collection of diseases that share a common characteristic. More than 200 types of cancer have been identified, affecting nearly every tissue in the body. The unifying feature that defines cancer is the uncontrolled proliferation of cells and tumour formation. The most common types of cancer in the UK are breast, lung, colorectal (bowel) and prostate cancer, which together account for more than half of all new cancer diagnoses (see **Figure 28**).[257]

Cancer incidence rates increased by 25 per cent in the UK in the past 40 years, but have stabilised over the past ten years (see **Figure 29**).[256] Part of this increase reflects longer life expectancy, and part is a result of lifestyle changes and the environment.[256] Cancer survival rates have doubled in the same time period; half of all people diagnosed with cancer will survive for five years or more.[256] There is significant variation in these figures, which are dependent on cancer type (site and cell type). In contrast to other cancers, lung cancer incidence and mortality has decreased over this period due almost exclusively to the reduction in smoking rates over the same period.[256]

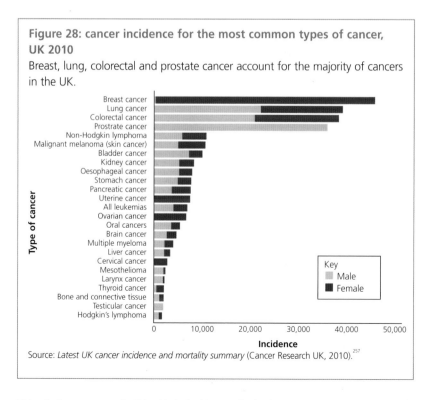

Figure 28: cancer incidence for the most common types of cancer, UK 2010

Breast, lung, colorectal and prostate cancer account for the majority of cancers in the UK.

Source: *Latest UK cancer incidence and mortality summary* (Cancer Research UK, 2010).[257]

Figure 29: cancer incidence and mortality, 1971-1999
Cancer incidence has increased since the 1970s, but advances in effective treatments have reduced mortality rates from cancer over the same period.

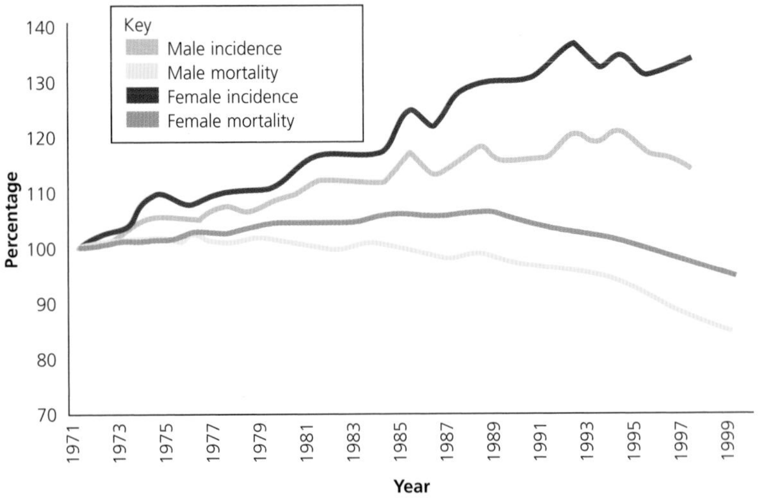

Key
Male incidence
Male mortality
Female incidence
Female mortality

Percentage / Year

Source: Cancer trends in England and Wales 1950-1999 (Office for National Statistics).[258]

What are the risk factors for developing cancer?
Lifestyle and environmental risk factors increase an individual's risk of cancer. These include tobacco and alcohol consumption, poor diet, overweight/obesity, physical inactivity, sun exposure (including the use of sunbeds) and unsafe sex. It is estimated that poor diet alone is associated with one quarter of all cancers (see **Box 10**).[152]

As outlined in the 2008 BMA Board of Science web resource *Cancer genetics*, cancer is not usually a hereditary disease. Fewer than 10 per cent of cancers are inherited – the BRCA1/2 genes being a rare exception. Inheritance of BRCA1/2 confers as high as an 80 per cent chance of developing primary breast cancer and 60 per cent of ovarian cancer.[259]

Cancer has a genetic element; mutations to genes occur in cells, which leads to an increased risk of abnormal cell proliferation and thus of tumour development. These occur in different cell lines and sites, but not in the germ line cells (sperm and ova), and are thus not inherited. The major factors affecting the development of mutation are the cellular environment, affected by lifestyle environmental and other factors. Environmental carcinogens include sun exposure, radiation, some viruses, certain chemicals and pesticides, and air and other pollution. Reproductive history, including age at first childbirth and number of children, can also affect the likelihood of some cancers in women.

Box 10 – diet and cancer

It is estimated that up to a quarter of the most common cancers can be prevented through changes to diet and physical activity levels.

The World Cancer Research Fund (WCRF) reviewed the evidence and medical literature surrounding the link between diet and cancer in 2007.[152] The report presented a list of foods and dietary habits that were either risk factors or protective factors for the most common cancers. The main findings are summarised below.

Risk Factors	*Protective Factors*
Red meat	Dietary fibre
Processed meat	Fruit
Salt and salty foods	Non-starchy vegetables
Fast food	Foods containing certain vitamins
Alcohol	Lactation and being breastfed
Overweight and obesity	Physical activity

Based on this review, the WCRF made a number of dietary recommendations to reduce the risk of cancer. The recommendations, as with the findings of the study, are compatible with findings from research studying the effects of diet on cardiovascular disease, diabetes and obesity.

To reduce cancer risk, the WCRF recommended that individuals:
- maintain a lean body weight
- limit consumption of high energy foods
- limit consumption of meat
- primarily eat plant-based foods
- limit alcohol consumption
- limit salt intake
- be physically active in everyday life
- breastfeed infants for at least six months.

The WCRF press release focused on the need to maintain a lean body weight, the contribution of red and processed meat to cancer risk, and the protective effects of breastfeeding. Communication of this message proved problematic. Researchers were clear that this was "good news"; lifestyle manipulations can very significantly reduce an individual's risk of developing a number of different cancers. The media portrayed it as a message that almost all foods were linked to cancer.

Summary

Cancer is a major cause of premature death in UK and high income countries worldwide. There are a number of known modifiable risk factors for cancer, including tobacco and alcohol use, poor diet, physical inactivity, sun exposure, unsafe sex, and overweight and obesity. There is scope to reduce the risk of developing cancer by increasing public awareness of these risk factors. Cancer remains primarily a disease of older age, and those under 60 years of age are at lower risk of cancer.

Further BMA resources:
- *Cancer genetics.* British Medical Association (2008).[260]
- *Health and ageing.* British Medical Association (2008).[261]

3.3.5. Diabetes risk

The prevalence of diabetes has increased significantly across the world, and is a particular burden in low and middle income countries, where 80 per cent of deaths from diabetes occur.[262] Diabetes prevalence is increasing steadily in these countries, and late detection and poor access to healthcare further contribute to the burden of disease. Approximately 285 million people worldwide have diabetes.[263]

The prevalence of diabetes in the UK is increasing; four per cent of the population – one in 25 – are living with diabetes. In 2009 there were 2.6 million people over 20 years old living with diabetes, compared to 1.4 million in 1996.[264] There are an estimated further 500,000 undiagnosed cases. Up to 11 per cent of all deaths in the UK can be attributed to diabetes.[264]

Diabetes is a disease resulting from poor regulation of blood glucose (sugar), which causes raised levels of blood glucose (hyperglycaemia) in the body. Chronic hyperglycaemia eventually causes damage to nerves and blood vessels. There are two variations of diabetes – types 1 and 2 – that have distinct causes and risk factors. Type 1 diabetes is less prevalent, is commonly diagnosed in childhood, and occurs when the pancreas is incapable of producing insulin – the hormone that controls blood glucose levels. In type 2 diabetes, the pancreas either does not produce a sufficient amount of insulin, or the body is not able to use the insulin that is produced, a phenomenon known as insulin resistance. Approximately 90 per cent of diabetes diagnoses are for type 2 diabetes.[262, 264]

Common factors that increase the risk of type 2 diabetes are overweight, obesity, high energy diets and physical inactivity. Weight management, a healthy diet and regular exercise are effective measures in reducing the risk of diabetes.[264-268] There is also evidence for a genetic component to diabetes risk. The increased risk of a sibling developing diabetes if their non-identical twin has been diagnosed is 10 per cent; in identical twins, who share the same genetic material, the equivalent increased risk is 90 per cent.[264] The BMA Board of Science report *Diabetes Mellitus* (2004) discusses in greater detail the epidemiology of and risk factors for diabetes.

Diabetes as a risk factor

Diabetes is also a risk factor for a number of conditions including cardiovascular disease and stroke, kidney failure, blindness, dementia and premature death.[114, 263, 269] Diabetes is the leading cause of blindness in the UK, where diabetics are 10 to 20 times more at risk than the general population.[264] A condition known as diabetic retinopathy affects up to 60 per cent of people diagnosed with diabetes within 20 years.[264]

Approximately half of deaths attributable to diabetes occur in those under 70 years of age – in contrast to other major diseases such as cardiovascular disease and cancer, which are typically diseases affecting older people.[264] The overall risk of premature death for people with diabetes is twice that compared to those without.[264] Average life expectancy is decreased by 10 years in type 2 diabetics, and over 20 years in type 1 diabetics.[264]

In the UK, 52 per cent of people with diabetes die from cardiovascular disease, predominantly heart disease and stroke. Diabetics are at twice the risk of stroke than the general population. Kidney failure is also common in those diagnosed with diabetes, where one in three type 2 diabetics will go on to develop kidney disease.[264, 268-269]

Summary

Prevalence of diabetes is increasing in the UK. Risk factors for developing type 2 diabetes include high energy diet, physical inactivity, and overweight and obesity. Diabetes itself is a risk factor for cardiovascular and renal diseases, and premature death.

> **Further BMA resources:**
> - *Diabetes mellitus: an update for healthcare professionals.* British Medical Association (2004).[269]

3.3.6. Dementia risk

The combination of an ageing population and increasing life expectancy means that the prevalence of dementia is set to increase rapidly in the UK. Dementia is the main cause of disability in old age and severely affects the ability to live independently.[270]

Dementia is a collection of diseases that affect the structure and chemistry of the brain, and lead to cognitive impairment and decline: loss of memory, communication and decision-making skills. These include Alzheimer's disease and vascular dementia, as well as rarer diseases such as vCJD and fronto-temporal dementia.

Dementia is common in the older population in the UK, and projected to more than double in the next 50 years.[271] The prevalence in the UK population is 1.1 per cent, but because it is an age-related disease, its prevalence is much higher in the older population, where five per cent of over-65s and 20 per cent of over-80s are diagnosed with a form of dementia (see **Figure 30**).[271] In the over-65s, prevalence of dementia doubles with every five years.[271] A more meaningful account of dementia risk is that in people who have survived to the age of 55, their remaining lifetime risk of developing dementia is 17 per cent in women and nine per cent in men.[271]

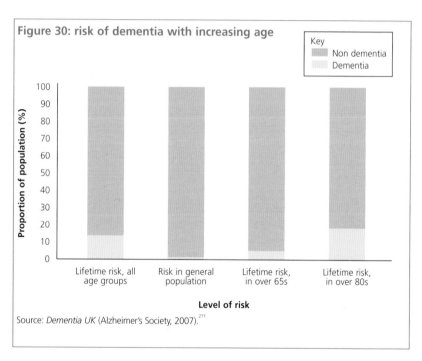

Figure 30: risk of dementia with increasing age

Key
■ Non dementia
▨ Dementia

Proportion of population (%)

Level of risk: Lifetime risk, all age groups / Risk in general population / Lifetime risk, in over 65s / Lifetime risk, in over 80s

Source: *Dementia UK* (Alzheimer's Society, 2007).[271]

There are several known risk factors for many types of dementia, of which age is the most significant. Lifestyle factors include high cholesterol, blood pressure and dietary fat intake,[272] physical and mental inactivity,[273-74] type 2 diabetes, atherosclerosis, and smoking.[272] Women are also more likely to develop dementia than men.[271] High fish consumption, educational attainment and vaccination against polio, diphtheria, tetanus or influenza are protective risk factors.[271-274]

The effect of inheritance and genetics in dementia is comparatively small. The incidence of parents or relatives living with dementia increases a person's risk of dementia only incrementally. For late-onset dementia, inheriting the gene variant APOE4 increases risk, although families carrying this gene variant are rare in the UK, and a relatively small proportion of people living with dementia carry this gene variant. Inheriting one copy of the APOE4 gene confers four times the risk of Alzheimer's disease than the general population, and inheriting two copies increases the risk ten fold. For the few people who carry this gene variant, this represents a high risk of developing dementia in later life – approximately a 20-50 per cent lifetime risk at the age of 65.[271, 275] Genetic inheritance and its associated risks are discussed in more detail in section 3.3.7.

Summary
The prevalence of dementia is set to increase rapidly in the UK in the next decades. Age is an important risk factor for dementia, but lifestyle and genetic risk factors are also associated with the disease. Dementia is primarily a disease of old age, and those under 65 years of age are at low risk of dementia.

Further BMA resources:
- *Health and ageing.* British Medical Association (2008).[261]

3.3.7. Genetic risk
Genetic risk is conceptually different from the other risks described in this report, as an individual's genetic make-up is uniquely personal. It is also, for the most part, fixed and not easily modified.

In humans, 99.7 per cent of DNA is common to all individuals. The remaining 0.3 per cent of genetic variation allows for substantial variation between individuals – in many physical traits from blood groups to hair, eye and skin colour. It may also confer substantial variation in susceptibility to disease.

Single gene disorders
If a genetic mutation is present in germ cells – sperm and ova – then it can be passed on to the next generation and inherited within families. If this type of genetic mutation interferes with the normal functioning of a gene in the body, it can cause illness. These types of illnesses are called single gene disorders – over 4,000 different disorders have been identified. Other types of hereditary genetic disorders involve structural variation, for example in Down's syndrome, which is a result of an extra copy of chromosome 21.

Although each genetic disorder is rare, collectively they occur in one to two per cent of the population.[276] While this population prevalence is relatively low, if an individual has a family history of a single gene disorder, their own and their children's risk of developing this disease increases significantly.

The inheritance pattern of a disorder has an influence on the risk of disease (see **Figure 31**). If the disorder is 'autosomal recessive', a person requires both copies of the mutant gene to develop the disease.[277-278] A person with one abnormal and one normal gene copy is a 'carrier'; they will not normally show signs of disease but can pass the mutation on to their children. If both parents are carriers of the genetic mutation, their children will each have a 25 per cent risk of inheriting two copies of the mutant gene and developing the disease.[277-278]

A common autosomal recessive disorder is cystic fibrosis. The disease is the result of mutations of the cystic fibrosis transmembrane regulator (CFTR) gene, which encodes for a protein involved in mucus production. Abnormal mucus production leads to the development of fibrosis and cysts in the lungs, and gastrointestinal illnesses. Approximately 40 per 100,000 infants born in the UK have cystic fibrosis, and there are currently approximately 7,500 people living with cystic fibrosis in the UK, of which 96.3 per cent are Caucasian.[279-280] Since 2003, the NHS UK Newborn Screening Programme offers genetic testing for all newborns for cystic fibrosis, as well as for congenital hypothyroidism, phenylketonuria, medium-chain acyl-CoA dehydrogenase deficiency (MCADD), sickle cell diseases and Tay Sachs disease (**see Box 11**). Early diagnosis enables earlier treatment with high energy diet, physiotherapy and medication, and can prolong life expectancy.[281]

If a disorder is 'autosomal dominant', an individual only requires one copy of the mutant gene to develop the disease.[277-278] This is the case with Huntington's disease, where if a parent has the disease, there is a 50 per cent chance that their children will also inherit the disease.[276, 282] Gene-environment interactions can influence the severity of a disease experienced by individuals with single-gene disorders (see page 97).

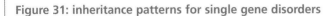

Figure 31: inheritance patterns for single gene disorders

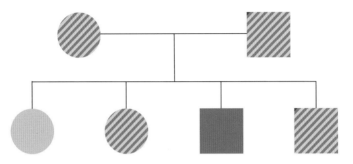

Autosomal recessive: pattern of inheritance when both parents are carriers of a recessive gene mutation

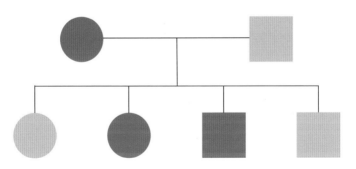

Autosomal dominant: pattern of inheritance when one parent is a carrier of a dominant gene mutations

 Normal   Carrier   Disease phenotype

Circle: female.   Square: male.

Source: *A guide to genetics* (Progress Educational Trust, 2006) and
Genetics home reference handbook (US National Library of Medicine, 2011).[277-278]

'Sex-linked' disorders result from mutations on the sex chromosomes (X and Y) and carry different genetic risk in males or females (see **Figure 32**). If a mother (who has two X chromosomes), is a carrier of a sex-linked genetic mutation on the X chromosome, her daughters have a 25 per cent chance of inheriting the mutation and being carriers, but her sons (who have only one X chromosome, always inherited from the mother) will have a 50 per cent chance of inheriting the mutation and developing disease. If the father is living with the genetic disorder, his daughters will have a 50 per cent chance of inheriting the mutation and being carriers, but his sons will not inherit the mutation because they will only inherit the Y chromosome. Examples of sex-linked genetic disorders include haemophilia and Duchene Muscular Dystrophy.[276-277, 282]

Figure 32: inheritance patterns for sex-linked gene disorders

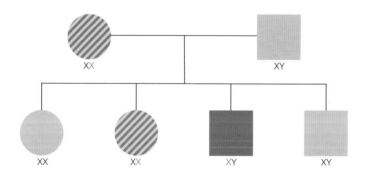

Pattern of inheritance when the mother is a carrier on the X chromosome

Source: *A guide to genetics* (Progress Educational Trust, 2006) and
Genetics home reference handbook (US National Library of Medicine, 2011).[277-278]

For single gene disorders, genetic testing results can affect knowledge about risk in two ways. A positive test result for a single gene disorder will indicate that an individual's risk of developing the disorder will be increased from 25 or 50 per cent to 100 per cent. A negative test result indicates that their risk is zero. The genetic test can be predictive or help to diagnose a latent disease.

A genetic test performed on an individual who knows there is an inheritable disease in their family may help them, alongside genetic counselling, to make reproductive choices, preventing the birth of more disease carriers or affected children (see **Box 11**).[276-277, 282]

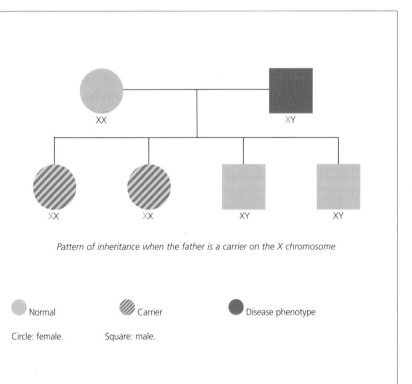

Pattern of inheritance when the father is a carrier on the X chromosome

Normal   Carrier   Disease phenotype

Circle: female.   Square: male.

Box 11: Tay Sachs Disease
Genetic testing, counselling, and awareness has led to the reduced prevalence of Tay Sachs disease in the Ashkenazi Jewish population.

Tay Sachs disease is an autosomal recessive disorder caused by a genetic mutation of the HEXA gene. This mutation results in the progressive destruction of nerve cells in the brain and spinal cord, causing deafness, blindness, loss of motor skills, delayed mental and social skills and premature death in children born with the disease. An individual is only affected when they inherit two mutant copies of the HEXA gene, one from each of their parents. Individuals with one normal copy of the HEXA gene and one abnormal copy are unaffected by the disease, but are carriers and have a 25 per cent chance of having an affected child (see **Figure 32**).[277]

Tay Sachs disease is known to be more prevalent in the Ashkenazi Jewish population than in other ethnic groups – affecting 0.4 individuals per 100,000 non-Jewish population, and 28 individuals per 100,000 in the Jewish population. Approximately 37 people per 1,000 in Jewish populations are carriers for the HEXA mutations that cause Tay Sachs disease, compared to four per 1,000 in the non-Jewish population.[283-284]

In the UK, community awareness projects, and the availability of genetic counselling and carrier testing for HEXA mutations has led to a 50 per cent reduction in the cases of Tay Sachs disease in the Jewish community since 2000.[283] In the US, awareness and genetic testing have also been successful in decreasing the prevalence of Tay Sachs disease by more than 90 per cent. As part of the screening programme, the initiatives have had a strong focus on education, genetic counselling, patient confidentiality and privacy. Since 1970, more than 1.4 million at-risk individuals have been screened for carrier status of the HEXA mutation, which has identified more than 1,400 couples at risk of having children with Tay Sachs Disease.[285]

Penetrance

Penetrance is used to describe the risk of disease for a given genetic mutation: the likelihood that a person with a given genetic mutation will go on to develop the associated disease. In many single gene disorders, the penetrance is effectively 100 per cent, for example with Huntington's disease and cystic fibrosis. In other mutations associated with more common diseases the penetrance is lower. The penetrance of the BRCA1 gene associated with breast cancer, for example, is 65 to 80 per cent[259] – not everyone with this genetic mutation will go on to develop breast cancer. For common diseases with complex genetic associations, penetrance is very low and as such has limited value in predicting risk of disease (see **Figure 33**).

Figure 33: penetrance and prevalence of selected gene variants
While the prevalence of a genetic variant associated with disease may be very low, the penetrance of the disease phenotype in individuals who inherit the gene variant can be very high, and vice versa.

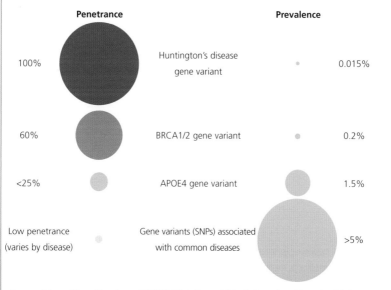

Source: Adapted from Hoppitt et al (2010), Manolio et al (2010), Scuteri et al (2010), *Alzheimer's disease* (POST, 2007), Esther et al (2007), and *Genetics – an overview* (PHG Foundation, 2006).[272, 286-288]

Even if the penetrance of a disease is high, its severity can vary between person to person. Although the penetrance of the gene for Huntington's disease is 100 per cent, the age of onset and disease progression varies from person to person. This may be dependent on other genetic and environmental factors interacting with the genetic mutation.

Genetic causes of common diseases

Almost all diseases have a genetic or hereditary component, however minor. The interaction of an individual's unique genetic makeup (their genome) with environmental and lifestyle factors may confer increased or decreased risk for certain diseases. It is not likely that a single gene will be responsible for this effect, but a combination of hundreds or thousands of genes each conferring incremental protection or vulnerability. These will have a cumulative effect of influencing the risk of disease. Caution is required in assuming that the 'hereditary' nature of some common diseases is genetic. While families share similar genetic risk factors, they also share many environmental and lifestyle risk factors.[276, 282]

Researchers identify the genetic influence of common diseases through genome-wide association studies (GWAS) – case-control studies that look for genetic variation between a group of individuals with a given condition (for example asthma), and a group of individuals without (the control group). The genetic variants are said to be 'associated' with the disease if they are observed statistically more often in the disease group than the control group. This approach is quite different to identifying genetic mutations with high penetrance in single gene disorders. There is typically significant overlap between control and disease groups that can only be differentiated using complex statistics.[287, 289-291]

Although GWAS have proved useful in understanding complex genetic disorders and the genetic basis of common diseases, in terms of disease risk prediction they are currently of little value. For most common diseases, the total hereditary component to disease risk is low, compared to the other environmental and lifestyle factors. Each individual genetic variant identified is only weakly associated with risk of disease, and the sum of the identified variants only account for a small proportion of the hereditary component of the disease.[287, 290] The genetic risk factors for many common diseases have not yet been fully identified, and only account for a small component of the disease risk.

Summary
Genetic makeup can predispose an individual to common and rare diseases.
Information from genetic testing may improve predictions of disease risk for
a variety of diseases in an individual. This information, where it relates to rare,
heritable diseases, may help individuals to make reproductive choices. In many
instances, however, knowledge of a genetic predisposition to a common disease
may be of little value without additional context, and because the genetic risk
cannot be modified.

Further BMA resources:
- *Population screening and genetic testing.* British Medical Association (2005).[292]

3.4.   Risks in healthcare

The previous section has reviewed the major diseases and the risk factors that
contribute to their development. For many of these diseases there are
technologies and medicines that can be used to treat, prevent or even cure
them. No treatment is risk-free. For all medical interventions, it is necessary
to balance the likelihood of improved health against the risk that the treatment,
or doing nothing, will cause harm.

For many diseases there are strategies including lifestyle changes and
preventative medicines that can decrease their likelihood in an individual.
But most people will suffer from illnesses of some sort, and have to make
treatment decisions.

Whether the medical condition is minor or major, life-threatening or not, acute
or chronic, the patient and their doctors will make treatment choices based
upon a series of options. They will balance the benefits from the treatment
with the costs, side effects, limitation on lifestyle, pain or discomfort, and risks
of serious sequelae with the consequences of alternative treatments or no
treatment. For every patient particular elements assume importance; these vary
between individuals. In some people being pain-free matters most, for others

being alert and able to interact with others. A 'cure' is not always the desired end point if the side effects of achieving it are too much for that patient.

Throughout the decision-making process the risks and benefits play an equally important part; doctors help patients to understand them and balance them within their options. Communicating these risks alongside the expected benefits is essential to gain informed consent to a treatment. Doctors can play an important role in helping patients put these risks in perspective.

3.4.1.   Medicines

Individual doctors cannot treat a sufficient number of patients with the same disease and treatment to be able to make quantitative assessments of the risks and benefits of the treatments they prescribe. They rely on research, principally RCTs, that can gather large amounts of data to assess the efficacy and risks associated with any treatment – pharmaceutical, surgical, diagnostic, or other.

Clinical trials are now a prerequisite for any new medicine, be it prescription or over-the-counter drugs. As highlighted in the 2005 BMA Board of Science report *Over the counter medication*, because clinical trials are conducted under strictly controlled conditions, translation to real clinical practice or over-the-counter availability may reveal additional risks associated with not following the prescription, using the drug in an unintended way, or pharmacological interactions with other drugs.[293] The British National Formulary (BNF) publishes information on reported side effects – minor and serious – for all licensed drugs in the UK. As highlighted in the first chapter, post-marketing surveillance is also an important mechanism for detecting adverse reactions.

The risk of a serious adverse drug reaction occurring is dependent on the drug, the patient's medical condition, and other lifestyle and genetic risk factors. When adverse reactions are extremely rare, a clinical trial would require hundreds of thousands of participants to detect these reactions, which is impractical, and costly, and would slow the introduction of a possibly valuable new agent to an unacceptable delay. Pharmacovigilance such as prescription event monitoring and the Yellow Card Scheme reports of adverse reactions are useful in bridging the gap between clinical trial information and anecdotal evidence. Where clinical trials have subsequently been conducted, they tend to agree with the anecdotally reported side effects. If an adverse reaction is already a very common condition – for example a headache – it may be difficult to establish the association statistically through clinical trials. The more widespread a drug's use, the greater the ability to detect these adverse reactions. The BMA Board of Science report *Reporting adverse drug reactions* (2006) discusses the effectiveness of these pharmacovigilance strategies in detecting rare risks in more detail.[8]

Summary
Prescription and over-the-counter medicines are routinely tested for safety, side effects and adverse reactions. This is in the form of clinical trials before licensing, and post-marketing surveillance and pharmacovigilance once approved for medical use. All medicines carry the risk of an adverse reaction. When used as directed, the benefits of medicines outweigh their risks.

Further BMA resources:
- *Evidence-based prescribing.* British Medical Association (2007).[294]
- *Over-the-counter medication.* British Medical Association (2007).[293]
- *Reporting adverse drug reactions: a guide for healthcare professionals.* British Medical Association (2006).[8]

3.4.2. Complementary and alternative medicine
A key concern with complementary and alternative medicine (CAM) is the scarcity of data to demonstrate the effectiveness and risks associated with CAM therapies. It appears that the treatments are less frequently subjected to controlled clinical trials or even monitoring, which are standard practice for conventional medical treatments.[295]

Although commonly perceived by the public as traditional and natural, therefore safe, CAM therapies carry risks, as with any treatment. Examples of possible harm include adverse effects from chiropractic treatment (including pain, stroke, and death),[296-297] infection and tissue trauma from acupuncture, liver and kidney toxicity from some herbal medicines, and allergic reactions to homeopathic treatments.[295] Some CAM therapies can also interact with conventional medicines, which may lead to health complications. The herbal medicine St John's wort is known to interact with, and reduce the effectiveness of, several conventional drugs, including the contraceptive pill, immunosuppressants, and anticoagulants.[298]

Even where there is a relatively low specific risk associated with the use of CAM, there is the additional risk that a patient may delay obtaining a definitive diagnosis until their condition has deteriorated to a point where allopathic treatment will be less effective.

The BMA has called for regulation of CAM treatments to the same standards expected of conventional medical treatments and procedures. Without evidence of clinical efficacy, it is impossible to assess the benefits and harms of the treatments. The BMA Board of Science also published the web resource *Complementary and alternative medicine: what your patients may be using* (2009) to support doctors in helping their patients make informed decisions about the use of CAM therapies.

Summary
As with conventional medicine, there are risks associated with the use of CAM therapies, such as adverse reactions. Some of these therapies may also cause harm through interactions with conventional medicines. In light of the absence of evidence demonstrating their effectiveness, there are additional risks associated with the use of CAM therapies, including that patients will delay seeking conventional medical treatment.

Further BMA resources:
- *Complementary and alternative medicine: what your patients may be using.* British Medical Association (2009).[299]

Paragraph 1, line 7
should not include
hepatitis C.

Erratum.

3.4.3.   Immunisation

Population immunisation is a preventive measure against future health risks, but there are also risks associated with the immunisation process. The reduction of future risk is far greater than the relatively minor risks of the immunisation procedure. Immunisation has been very effective in preventing a number of diseases, including the worldwide eradication of smallpox and the significant reduction in prevalence of polio, diphtheria, pertussis, measles, mumps, rubella, meningitis, and hepatitis B and C. The fragility of these success stories is shown by the increase in epidemic measles in Western Europe in late 2010 and early 2011, coinciding with decreased immunisation levels in the population.[300]

The principle of immunisation is that to lower or eliminate the risk of disease in the population in the future, a person incurs a small risk from the immunisation process. This risk is very low – in particular when compared to the risk and consequence of the diseases that they prevent – and can include temporary pain, headache, nausea, vomiting, or mild fever.

At the population level, immunisation of the majority against a particular disease will reduce the prevalence of disease by limiting its ability to infect and spread. This concept of 'herd immunity' requires that individuals in a population incur a small increased risk of ill-health from immunisation in order to benefit from population immunity against a communicable disease – thereby reducing the risk of infection and disease in the whole population.

Immunisation rates in the UK are high. Uptake of vaccines against diphtheria, tetanus, polio, pertussis, and meningitis C is approximately 94 per cent in infants.[301] As noted in the first chapter, the uptake of the vaccine against MMR is lower at 89 per cent (see pages 26-27). Uptake of the vaccine against the human papilloma virus, which protects against cervical cancer, is at 70 per cent among 12 to 13 year old girls.[301-302]

Many immunisation programmes are targeted at infants and young children, and require parental consent. Parents are very protective of the health and safety of their children, avoiding any perceived risks to their child, and acting in what they believe are the child's best interests. In communicating with parents, health professionals should address the concerns of parents in a transparent and open manner.[303] While the risks about which parents express concern may not have validity or evidence base, healthcare professionals must understand their basis in the parents' belief system. They should be open and honest about the benefits of immunisation to the child and the community, and to any of the parents' other (future) children.

Summary
The benefits of immunisation greatly outweigh the risks to the population. Public anxiety surrounding vaccination can have a real impact on immunisation levels and lead to an increase in infection rates. As immunisation programmes often focus on children, the perception of risk can be heightened. Many people may be reluctant to participate in immunisation programmes because the immediate risk of harm from the vaccination procedure is perceived as greater than the future risk of infection.

Further BMA resources:
- *Childhood immunisation: a guide for healthcare professionals.* British Medical Association (2003).[304]

3.4.4. Screening
Screening tests are population-level preventive measures that can be used to predict an individual's future risk of disease and allow them to take measures to minimise their risk factors before they cause illness. Decisions about screening uptake can be influenced by the risk information communicated to the patient. Patients provided with individually tailored risk information are more likely to undergo screening tests than patients presented with average population risk information.[305]

As highlighted in the 2005 BMA Board of Science report *Population screening and genetic testing*, screening tests, and any follow up tests, carry risks, which can be significant. Many tests are invasive, uncomfortable or involve a radiation dose. Follow up tests and preventive measures can include further invasive procedures and surgery. For those who benefit from early detection, these risks are considered minimal compared to the benefits of early detection and treatment.

When screening an asymptomatic population, there is a high probability of false positive test results. Even if the specificity of the screening test (the ability to correctly identify the individuals who do not have the disease) is high at 95 per cent, the majority of positive test results will be false positive. This is because the prevalence of the disease being screened for in the general population is typically lower than five per cent. These false positive results may expose individuals to the unnecessary risks of follow-up treatments.

For some diseases, including some cancers, there is an additional risk of overdiagnosis from screening tests: the diagnosis of disease that would not have become clinically apparent during a patient's lifetime. In this case, the disease is correctly diagnosed (true positive) but would not have caused illness or death in the patient if undetected. Overdiagnosis as a result of screening leads to overtreatment of disease, which has associated harms.

Using mammography breast cancer screening as an example, the flow chart in **Figure 34** describes the likelihoods of true positive (cancer diagnosis), true negative (no diagnosis), false negative (undiagnosed cancer) and false positive (diagnosis in healthy women) results in a group of 1,000 women. For every seven women correctly diagnosed with breast cancer, 70 healthy women will receive a positive test result and require further tests, and one woman with breast cancer will go undiagnosed.[306] A recent study estimated that up to one in three breast cancer diagnoses from mammography screening were overdiagnosed.[307] In this example, in approximately two of the seven women correctly diagnosed with cancer, the cancer would not otherwise have become clinically apparent in their lifetime.

Mammography screening was introduced in the UK in 1988, and at present, the UK National Screening Committee (NSC) considers that the benefits of breast cancer screening in women aged 50 to 70 outweigh the harms. At present the NSC recommends screening in this group (see page 103), but this recommendation is currently under review.[308] As screening and early detection improves outcomes in women with cancer, the harms of follow-up tests for women with false positive test results (eg further radiation exposure) are deemed acceptable.

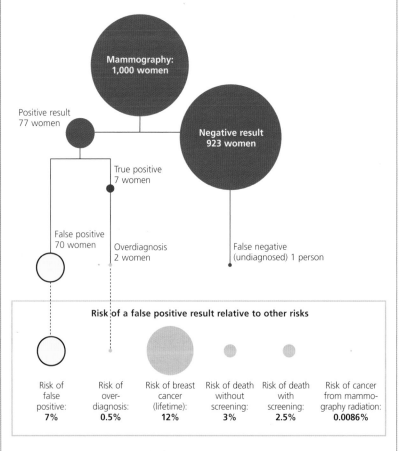

Figure 34: risks associated with mammography screening for breast cancer.
The risks of false positive and false negative diagnoses are acceptable relative to the risks of breast cancer incidence and mortality, and the risks of mammography itself.

Mammography:
1,000 women

Positive result
77 women

Negative result
923 women

True positive
7 women

False positive
70 women

Overdiagnosis
2 women

False negative
(undiagnosed) 1 person

Risk of a false positive result relative to other risks

| Risk of false positive: **7%** | Risk of over-diagnosis: **0.5%** | Risk of breast cancer (lifetime): **12%** | Risk of death without screening: **3%** | Risk of death with screening: **2.5%** | Risk of cancer from mammo-graphy radiation: **0.0086%** |

Source: Adapted from *Breast cancer facts* (Cancer Research UK, 2010), Gotzsche et al (2011), Gigerenzer et al (2003), Tabar et al (2000) and Jorgensen et al.[50, 79, 306-307]

For any screening test, the potential benefits of the test must be balanced against its associated risks. These risks should be communicated to patients alongside the intended benefits of the screening test, to enable informed patient choice. There is some concern that information communicated to patients about NHS screening programmes does not always adequately discuss the risks of false positive and negative results, and of overdiagnosis. Some healthcare professionals have begun to question whether the benefit of early detection of breast cancer in a small proportion of screened women truly outweighs the harms associated with overdiagnosis and false positive results from mammography screening. The 10-year survival rates for women with breast cancer if they are screened or not screened are similar – 90.25 and 90.20 per cent, respectively.[79, 309] The risks as well as the potential benefits of breast cancer screening should be clearly communicated to patients by healthcare professionals, rather than only the intended benefits.[309]

Amniocentesis during pregnancy is another example of a screening test that may be indicated in some pregnant women. The procedure involves inserting a fine gauge needle through the abdomen and into the womb, and collecting a small volume of amniotic fluid. The fluid contains fetal cells that can be tested to diagnose a range of genetic conditions, including Down's syndrome, Edward's syndrome, and other inherited genetic disorders such as Duchene Muscular Dystrophy, haemophilia, thalassaemia or sickle cell anaemia.

Women who are over 35 years of age, have a family history of a genetic disorder, or are at increased risk of having a baby with Down's syndrome, are offered amniocentesis at 15 weeks. A negative diagnosis confirms that the fetus is free from the genetic disorder. A positive diagnosis can help women decide whether to terminate the pregnancy or, if they choose to continue the pregnancy, prepare to support their child with a genetic disorder. The procedure itself carries a one in 100 risk of subsequent miscarriage, and a one in 1,000 risk of infection, which may lead to complications in the pregnancy.[310] Pregnant women offered amniocentesis need to balance the risks of the procedure with the benefits of genetic testing, which include family planning and reproductive choices.[310-311]

UK National Screening Committee

The NSC reviews available and future screening tests to determine whether screening should be offered based on defined criteria such as clinical validity of any screening test, benefits and harms, and cost effectiveness. More than 100 screening tests have been reviewed by the NSC, including antenatal and newborn screening, child health, STIs, cancer, and vascular diseases.

Many screening tests have not been recommended by the NSC, because the risks of screening outweigh the potential benefits in the general population. The prostate specific antigen (PSA) test for prostate cancer is not recommended by the NSC because it has a high false positive and false negative rate.

Direct-to-consumer screening tests

Tests not recommended by the NSC or offered through the NHS may be available through private healthcare services and marketed directly to the public. In very rare cases, new and effective screening tests are available privately before being recommended by the NSC (eg abdominal aortic aneurism screening, which is being introduced in the NHS after a 2009 recommendation by the NSC). In some cases the tests on offer privately are either not effective at predicting disease risk, have high false positive or negative rates, or there are no effective measures to reduce risk if a positive result is found.

In June 2010, the BMA and the Academy of Medical Royal Colleges (AoMRC) published a joint statement calling on the UK Government to strengthen existing regulation surrounding direct-to-consumer screening tests. Companies offering tests should be required to provide factual and balanced information to consumers on the risks and limitations associated with the test, the implications of the results, and any follow up that might be required.

Summary

Screening is intended to benefit patient health through early detection of disease. Screening procedures themselves have associated risks, and the potential benefits of screening must be balanced against these risks. Screening in an asymptomatic population has a high likelihood of false diagnosis, even when tests are highly specific. Communication of the risks and benefits of screening tests is essential to ensure informed patient consent.

> **Further BMA resources:**
> - *Joint statement on direct-to-consumer screening.* British Medical Association (2010).[312]
> - *Population screening and genetic testing.* British Medical Association (2005).[292]

3.4.5.   Surgery

Surgery describes a series of physical interventions that change the anatomy of the individual. The aim is to remove, alter or adjust an anatomical element that is causing illness and thus to alleviate or cure that illness – prolonging and improving the quality of life.

Surgery has specific and general risks associated with it. General risks pertain to all surgical procedures – although at different levels of likelihood and severity – and include premature death, haemorrhage, infection, and disability.

Over the last century surgery has become safer due to increased understanding and improvement in surgical practice. Death from general anaesthesia remains a risk of surgery, but has been significantly reduced in recent decades with improvements in anaesthetic practice, agents, equipment, and monitoring systems. These improvements have led to an incidence of peri-operative death which can be directly attributable to anaesthesia from one in 6,795 (14.7 per 100,000 patients) in the 1950s, to one in 200,200 (0.5 per 100,000 patients) by the 1990s.[313]

The benefits of surgery are dependent on the underlying disease/condition, proposed procedure, patient lifestyle factors, and associated co-morbidities of the patient. The risks and potential complications of surgery will be dependent on individual risk factors, including age, lifestyle and co-morbidities, the proposed procedure or technique, the equipment, and the expertise of the surgeon. The benefits and risks of surgery are based on published results of case series or trials, and a hospital's surgery unit or an individual surgeon's own results.

Summary
The risks associated with surgery and the level of potential harm is dependent on the nature of the surgical procedure. Surgeons aim to ensure that for individual patients, the benefits of a surgical procedure outweigh the harms.

3.4.6.   Blood transfusion and the use of blood products

Modern blood transfusions and blood donation services were pioneered during the first and second World Wars, and have saved countless lives since, in particular in the treatment of trauma patients and for cases of life-threatening haemorrhage.[314] There were more than 117,000 blood transfusion procedures in England, Wales and Northern Ireland in 2010.[315] Blood transfusion has now become widespread in surgical practice and critical care, and are used in approximately half of the 30,000 cardiac operations that take place in the UK each year.[316] There are, however, a number of risks associated with blood transfusion, including allergic reaction, anaphylaxis (severe allergic reaction), infection, transfusion-related acute lung injury (TRALI), transfusion-associated circulatory overload (TACO) and incorrect blood component transfused (IBCT).[317]

The body's immune system may react to antibodies or other substances in donated blood, causing an allergic reaction. In 2010, there were 34 suspected cases of anaphylaxis following a blood transfusion in the UK, of which two contributed to the death of the patient. There were 15 reported cases of TACO causing severe morbidity or death. A medical emergency can result if a patient is mistakenly given the wrong blood type during a transfusion (IBCT). In 2010, there were two cases of IBCT in the UK, neither of which were fatal.[317]

The risk of bacterial or viral infection from donated blood is low, and there is a strict screening process for bacteria and viruses such as HIV, hepatitis B and C in the UK blood services. There have been no reported cases of viral infection from a blood transfusion since 2005. There were two confirmed cases of bacterial infection leading to sepsis following blood transfusion in 2009 in the UK (NHS) and none reported in 2010.[317]

Although there are no available blood tests to detect the presence of prions that contribute to the development of vCJD at present, only three cases of transmission of vCJD prions from donor to patient via blood transfusion have been reported, in each case blood transfusion occurred between 1996 and 1999.[318] Given the uncertainty surrounding the relationship between exposure to prions and the risk of developing vCJD, and the lack of any measures to prevent or delay the onset of the disease, the BMA highlighted ethical issues surrounding informing patients of their potential exposure to vCJD prions through medical procedures such as surgery and blood transfusion. A balance must be achieved between public health interests and the interests of the patient. While informing patients of their potential exposure could in theory minimise future risks to others from affected individuals, there also exists a risk of considerable psychological harm to the patient and an absence of any benefit to them at present from knowing of their potential exposure.[319]

Similarly, in the case of blood donation, the BMA's view is that, should a blood test for the detection of vCJD prions become available and required for blood donation, donors should be given the option of not receiving their test results, in the absence of any direct benefit to the patient and the risk of psychological harm.[319]

Blood transfusion may also be associated with increased mortality and morbidity following some surgical procedures such as cardiac or general surgery, and critical care. Some have questioned whether the potential benefits of blood transfusion outweigh it's risks for many procedures, with the exception of haemorrhagic shock where the benefits are substantial and life-saving.[314] A recent study estimated that the risk of death within a year of a cardiac surgery operation was three times greater in patients who received blood than in patients who did not, and experienced a threefold increase in heart attacks, stroke and renal failure.[316]

3.4.7. Healthcare-associated infections

Healthcare-associated infections (HCAIs) are the infections acquired within healthcare settings, including MRSA, *C. difficile*, and other less common agents. The infections can cause harm particularly in patients who may already be seriously ill or immune-compromised. Complications can include extended stays in hospital, pain, disability, or be a contributing factor to a patient's premature death. The BMA Board of Science reviewed the prevalence of HCAIs in the UK and strategies to mitigate HCAI transmission in hospital settings in its 2009 report *Taking action on healthcare associated infections* and its 2006 report *Healthcare associated infections – a guide for healthcare professionals*.

Patients are most at risk of infection following invasive procedures, including surgery, catheterisation, the introduction of intravenous devices, and artificial ventilation. The most common sites of HCAIs are gastrointestinal, urinary tract, surgical site, skin or soft tissue, or bloodstream. The risk of acquiring MRSA or *C. difficile* while in hospital is now declining, after intensive efforts to control infection.

What is the risk of HCAIs when accessing healthcare services?
Approximately eight to nine per cent of patients acquire a HCAI while accessing secondary (hospital) healthcare services – over 300,000 infections per year in the UK.[320] The incidence in the UK is high relative to other European countries. Although prevalence of all HCAIs has remained relatively static over the past decade, investment in prevention measures and mandatory surveillance for specific infections have resulted in a reduction of MRSA bloodstream infection and *C. difficile* reports in NHS Trusts since 2006.[321]

The DH in England estimates that up to 30 per cent of these infections are preventable, through adequate hand-washing and environmental hygiene, minimising infection from invasive procedures, and protective clothing.[322] Even with adequate measures to minimise the risk, 70 per cent cannot be prevented by improved hygiene. The prevalence of HCAIs is much lower in primary and community healthcare settings due to the nature of care – fewer invasive procedures are undertaken outside the hospital setting.

Mortality from HCAIs is decreasing. In 2010, there were 2,704 deaths from *C. difficile* in England and Wales – a prevalence of 2.57 per 100,000 population among males and 2.54 per 100,000 population among females.[323] There were 485 deaths from MRSA, which is a prevalence of 0.37 per 100,000 population in men and 0.37 per 100,000 population in women.[324]

Summary
While the lifetime risk of dying from a HCAI is low, the risk of acquiring a HCAI during a hospital visit in the UK is high relative to other European countries. The risk of infection is dependent on the nature of the visit, the procedures involved, and the patient's health. Measures have been identified that can reduce the risk of infection, but HCAIs are not entirely preventable.

3.4.8. Antimicrobial resistance

Antimicrobial resistance is an increasing risk. The use of antimicrobial drugs to treat infection is a defining feature of modern medicine. Their widespread use and misuse is causing the development of resistance. For every licensed antibiotic drug, there already exists a strain of resistant bacteria. The WHO estimates that within ten years, some diseases may have no effective therapies.[326]

Bacteria can rapidly acquire drug resistance because they can share genetic information, including genes for drug resistance, among and across bacterial strains. Excessive use of antimicrobial drugs in healthcare creates an environment where strains that have acquired resistance can flourish and replace strains that remain susceptible to the drugs.

The use of antibiotics in agriculture may contribute to the development of antimicrobial resistant strains of bacteria. Antibiotics are administered to animals with bacterial infections, and as a preventive measure against infection. Human exposure to antibiotic residues from milk and dairy products may lead to the development of antibiotic-resistant gut bacteria. These bacteria may in turn confer resistance to other more harmful bacteria.

Infection control becomes difficult where there are no effective antibiotics. The risk of spreading the infection is increased, as are the effects of infection in patients. In the UK, up to 14 per cent of cases of invasive pneumococci are resistant to the antimicrobial drug erythromycin, and two to four per cent are resistant to penicillin.[327-328] The number of cases of antibiotic-resistant tuberculosis has almost doubled in the UK between 2000 and 2009, from 206 cases to 389.[327] Globally, multi-drug resistant (MDR) and extensively drug resistant (XDR) tuberculosis are also becoming more prevalent.

Summary
Antimicrobial resistance is a significant issue for the control of infectious disease. The inappropriate use of antimicrobials increases the risk of resistant bacteria. At least one strain of resistant bacteria exist for every antimicrobial drug. The WHO predicts that some diseases may have no effective antimicrobial treatment within ten years.

3.4.9.   Medical technologies

Other medical technologies expose patients to increased risk, for example imaging techniques that require radiation exposure such as X-ray, positron emission tomography (PET), and computed tomography (CT). The risk is offset by the benefits of diagnosis and early treatment. If used to screen an asymptomatic population the risks of radiation exposure would be likely to exceed any benefit. This is illustrated by the use of whole-body CT scanning. This is a valuable diagnostic tool, but as recommended by the Committee on the Medical Aspects of Radiation in the Environment (COMARE), should be avoided for population screening.[329]

New medical technologies may present new types of risk about which there are higher levels of uncertainty. Regenerative medicine, stem cell therapy and tissue engineering have the potential to regenerate or replace damaged tissues and organs in the human body, but the risks of immune system reactions, cancer development and genetic interactions are not yet well characterised. These technologies are subject to the same level of regulation, risk assessment and management as other types of treatments before use in patients.

Summary
For every application, the benefits of medical technologies, including new technologies, should outweigh their risks. While CT scanning is a useful diagnostic tool, for example, its potential harms are greater than its benefits in the case of population screening.

3.4.10. Not seeking treatment

There are risks associated with not seeking treatment or delaying treatment. For many illnesses, early detection and intervention increases the chances of effective treatment and survival. Early detection of malignancies such as melanoma, breast, colorectal, cervical and lung cancer can increase the likelihood of long-term survival.[256, 330] Children and other vulnerable groups can also be at increased risk of poor health if their parent, guardian or carer delays or neglects to seek treatment on their behalf.

There are a number of recognised barriers to seeking treatment, including a lack of awareness of the signs and symptoms of cancer, emotional and practical barriers (eg too scared or worried, or too busy to seek treatment), as well as service barriers, in booking timely and convenient appointments.[330] The greater these perceived barriers, the more likely an individual will delay seeking treatment.[331]

Certain groups are less likely to seek treatment, including men, young people, individuals from low socioeconomic status groups and some ethnic minorities.[332] Men have been found, for example, to visit their general practitioner (GP) 20 per cent less frequently than women, for a range of common health conditions.[333]

For other conditions such as stroke, early recognition of symptoms and rapid treatment can help reduce brain damage and improve the chances of a full recovery. The importance of acting quickly when a stroke is suspected was highlighted by the 2008 Stroke Association 'FAST' campaign. This aimed to raise awareness of the symptoms of stroke: 'if someone is displaying symptoms of **f**acial weakness, **a**rm weakness or **s**peech problems, then it is **t**ime to call 999'.

Summary

Every medicine and medical procedure carries risks, but not seeking treatment also has its risks. Delayed treatment can exacerbate illness and reduce available treatment options. In avoiding potential harms of medical treatment, patients may expose themselves to other risks.

3.5.   Risk and the environment

The environment presents a number of risks to human health, from man-made and natural causes. Risks in the environment are often perceived to be beyond an individual's personal control, or of potentially catastrophic consequence, and therefore tend to be perceived as higher risk than some of the more common everyday lifestyle risks presented in the previous sections.

This section will outline some of the common sources of health risk associated with the environment, including chemical hazards, toxic waste and land contamination, radiation, disasters and emergencies, climate change, and extreme threats (such as terrorism).

3.5.1.   Chemical hazards

Individuals are exposed to and come into contact with thousands of chemicals in their daily lives. Many of these are essential for modern life – including plastics, which are widely used in many medical procedures, from syringes to prosthetic limbs, as well as chemicals used in building materials, food production and distribution. Many are also less toxic or damaging than the material they replace (eg a range of new chemicals in cosmetics have replaced heavy metals). Many chemicals are known to pose a risk to human health. These range from metals (including lead and mercury), organic compounds (including benzene, dioxins, and pesticides), to asbestos, arsenic and many other chemicals found in common household and beauty products, and as a component of air pollution from the combustion of fossil fuels.[334]

Every chemical, at sufficiently high dose, is toxic and has the potential to cause harm to health. The health harms from chemicals can range from respiratory, cardiovascular, digestive, skin and blood-related diseases, to autoimmune and endocrine diseases, congenital abnormalities, developmental disorders, and cancer.[3, 335]

With technological improvements, it is possible to detect minute concentrations of chemicals in products, the environment and in the human body. Determining acceptable levels of chemical exposure is necessary to manage the health risks. Chemical exposure in the public is relatively low and does not present a significant health risk.[334] Over a lifetime, the saturated fat, sugar and salt present in most processed foods pose a far greater risk than the chemical preservatives and colourants they contain. Those working in chemical, industrial or agricultural industries and who are exposed to higher chemical concentrations are most at risk.[3, 335]

The WHO estimates that the health harms from exposure to chemicals leads to 4.9 million deaths and 86 million DALYs per year. Approximately half of this burden of disease is borne by children younger than 15 years of age. Seventy per cent of the burden of disease is attributable to the chemicals present in air pollution, from road traffic emissions, and indoor pollutants from solid fuel combustion. A gradient exists in which lower income countries and the poorest in society are disproportionately affected. Occupational exposure, acute poisonings and pesticides account for 800,000 deaths per year worldwide.[334]

Summary
Over a lifetime, individuals may be exposed to thousands of chemicals as part of everyday life. Most chemicals pose a low risk of harm at normal levels of exposure, but chronic or significant exposure to certain chemicals can be a health risk.

3.5.2.   Toxic waste, land and water contamination
Chemical manufacture, industrial processes and sewage treatment produce large volumes of toxic waste, and their disposal and storage are environmental hazards and health hazards. The health risks of toxic waste include water and land contamination, which can cause poisoning and injury in neighbouring communities. These health risks can be amplified when toxic waste is exported to developing countries with less regulatory oversight of these industries and poor risk management practices.

Poor nuclear waste management practices can result in radioactive waste pollution into bodies of water and radon gas released into the atmosphere. Rather than being diluted in water systems, under some conditions it is concentrated within the marine food chain and can reach significant levels in large fish. It is estimated that the solid waste product will remain radioactive for 80,000 years, so reprocessing, accumulation and storage is an important aspect of nuclear energy risk management.[94] Identifying safe sites should therefore consider geopolitical, geological and climactic factors.

Minimising exposure to an industrial hazard in one group may mean increasing exposure to the hazard in another. This double standard occurs through industry exploiting regulatory weaknesses in developing countries. It is in contrast to what would be accepted in the developed country where the company is registered, or where a company faces pressure from well-informed and resourced local activists.[4]

This practice is known as the export of hazard, including toxic waste disposal practices or high risk labour conditions and machinery. The communities in developing countries to where the activity has been transferred are often not aware of the severity or nature of the hazard, and lack the resources, experience and resilience to respond to the hazard. The risk-benefit equation in these cases is distorted because the majority of the benefits of the activity are not transferred to the host community and remain in the developed countries.[4] The host community typically benefits only from (high risk) employment. The most devastating example of an incident where the export of hazard resulted in significant harm to local communities is the chemical and gas leak at the American company Union Carbide's pesticide factory in Bhopal, India in 1984. This claimed more than 10,000 thousand lives and caused several tens of thousands of injuries.[336]

Summary
If they are not properly managed and disposed of, the waste products associated with manufacturing, industry and energy can be a health risk to employees and neighbouring communities.

3.5.3.   Radiation
Radioactivity, in the form of alpha, beta, gamma or x rays, increases the risk of cancer, congenital birth defects and miscarriage. In high doses – which are extremely rare and typically the result of exposure from nuclear war or industrial disasters – it can cause radiation sickness and death.

In the UK, the public perception is that the greatest risks of radiation are from nuclear power plants and the radioactive waste it produces, followed by the threat of nuclear war.[337-339] In fact, the major source of radiation in the UK is in the form of radon gas which is present in the rock and soil in the ground, particularly in the southwest of England and in Scotland. In poorly ventilated homes, radon gas can accumulate to high levels and increase the lifetime risk of cancer.[340] Other important sources of radiation include medical sources and cosmic radiation (see **Figure 35**). The overall contribution of radon, and radiation in general, to the total cancer incidence is relatively low – approximately two per cent of cancers worldwide.[340]

Figure 35: the main sources of exposure to ionising radiation in the UK population
The majority (84%) of exposure to radiation is from natural sources. Exposure to artificial radiation (blue) is predominantly from medical sources of ionising radiation such as X-rays, CT and PET.

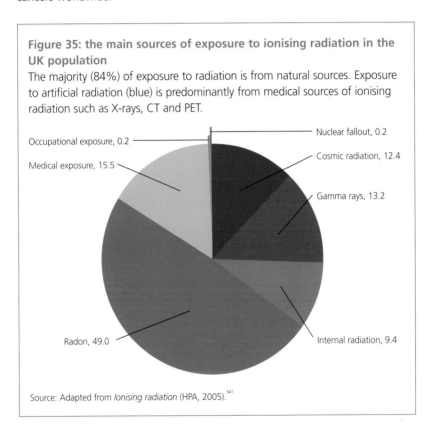

Occupational exposure, 0.2
Nuclear fallout, 0.2
Medical exposure, 15.5
Cosmic radiation, 12.4
Gamma rays, 13.2
Radon, 49.0
Internal radiation, 9.4

Source: Adapted from *Ionising radiation* (HPA, 2005).[341]

Current radiation protection legislation is based on the controversial 'linear no-threshold' (LNT) hypothesis. This states that risk from radiation continues proportionally down to even very low exposures, so that there is no threshold level of radiation exposure below which could be considered of negligible risk. Assuming the LNT hypothesis, the 70,000,000 CT scans carried out in the US in 2007 will lead to an estimated 29,000 cancers.[93, 342]

Low dose x-ray scanners are increasingly used at airport security stations. Known as backscatter scanners, a very low dose of radiation is used to image superficial soft tissue such as skin, and detect explosives or other devices hidden on the body. Apart from the privacy concerns of this technology, there are concerns surrounding the health harms of repeated exposure to x-rays in frequent flyers and air passengers in general.

A 2011 study attempted to quantify the radiation exposure and associated health risks of backscatter x-ray scanners to frequent flyers[h] and all flyers.[195] This concluded that the additional health risk posed from the scanners was negligible compared to current levels of natural and artificial exposure to radiation. The study estimated that 50 backscatter x-ray scans would be the equivalent of one dental radiograph, and more than 4,000 scans equivalent to one mammogram.[195] The risk of cancer from different forms of aviation-related radiation is described in **Table 5**.

Table 5 – risk of cancer from aviation-related radiation

	All flyers	Frequent flyers
Global population of passengers (estimate)	100,000,000	1,000,000
Cancers that would occur during a lifetime, from non-aviation causes	40,000,000	400,000
Cancers attributed to cosmic radiation exposure from flying	n/a	600
Cancers attributed to backscatter x-ray scanners	6	4

Source: *Mehta et al* (2011)[195]

Radiation exposure from nuclear power stations
The risk of massive leakage from failing nuclear reactors is widely recognised, potentially catastrophic and engineered against. Risk management procedures within nuclear power plants are stringent. Under normal operating conditions very little radioactive material escapes. Even if risk management strategies are able to

---

h A frequent flyer was defined as an individual (passenger, pilot or airline staff) who spend more than 60 hours flying per week over one year.

achieve a low overall risk, the consequences are major if an event does occur, as at Chernobyl in 1986 (see **Box 12**), and more recently the crisis at the Fukushima nuclear reactors in Japan in March 2011.

Box 12 – Chernobyl disaster 1986

The explosion of a nuclear reactor at the Chernobyl power station led to a massive release of ionising radiation – more than 6.7 tonnes of radioactive material – from the reactor core into the atmosphere. The radiation dispersed across a large area of Europe and the states of the former Soviet Union – a geographical spread of more than 200,000 square kilometres. Initial reports of the disaster were denied and then downplayed by the Russian authorities, and conflicting advice regarding food safety and travel within Europe created confusion and anxiety among the public.[343] The health effects of radiation dose to emergency workers and residents of affected communities have been studied closely since.

Emergency and clean-up workers

Emergency workers at the site received the highest doses of radiation – 134 were diagnosed with acute radiation sickness, and 28 died within four months of the disaster.[344] The fatality rate from acute radiation sickness of emergency workers who received doses in excess of six grays (Gy; 21 workers) was 95 per cent, and 32 per cent in those who received doses in excess of four Gy (134 workers).[345-347]

The majority of clean-up workers were exposed to less than 0.15 Gy and did not suffer radiation sickness. Radiation is known to concentrate in the thyroid, and average radiation dose to this organ was 0.21 Gy.[343-344, 346] To put this exposure in context, the radiation dose is approximately 100 times greater than the average annual exposure to ionising radiation in the UK population, and 30 times greater than an average CT brain scan.

Subsequent studies have shown that clean-up workers were at increased risk of leukaemia and thyroid cancer. The dose-dependent increased risk was similar to an earlier estimate from survivors of the atomic bombs in Hiroshima and Nagasaki in Japan.[345-347]

Neighbouring communities

In communities affected by elevated radiation exposure, a dose-dependent increased risk of thyroid cancer was observed in children, which was attributed to milk contaminated with Iodine-131, but no conclusive evidence exists for an increase in childhood leukemias.[346-347] More than 5,000 cases of thyroid cancer were reported in children in the five years following the disaster, but fewer than 20 of these children died.[343-344] The International Commission on Radiological Protection estimated that the Chernobyl disaster would result in 1,000 excess deaths in Western Europe, 1,250 in eastern Europe and 7,500 in the former Soviet Union during the subsequent 50 years. While these deaths are significant, they represent a small proportion of all deaths over this period.[345-347] The psychological effects on affected communities were, and continue to be, significant.[343-344]

In the wake of the Chernobyl disaster, many lessons were learned and safety improvements implemented on existing and newly-commissioned nuclear reactors. The reactors at the nuclear power plant at Fukushima in Japan were built in the 1970s. The magnitude 9.0 earthquake immediately triggered the automatic shutdown of all reactors. The tsunami that followed caused the backup generators that maintained the water cooling system to fail, leading to heating of the nuclear reactor cores. This resulted in a partial meltdown of the core, explosions in two of the four reactors, and release of nuclear material into the environment.

The importance of transparent and trusted communications, and rapid monitoring was stressed following the Chernobyl disaster.[343] The Japan Atomic Industrial Forum strived to publish daily updates on the Fukushima plant, and the international community closely monitored the situation. Longitudinal studies of the potential health effects to residents and power plant employees were rapidly established. In response to the leak, a 20km radius exclusion zone was designated around the power plant, and 80,000 residents were urged to leave the area. A further 136,000 residents in the 20-30km band were also advised to consider leaving their homes. Residents were urged to stay indoors as much as possible to avoid exposure to radiation, and potassium iodide tablets were distributed (to saturate the thyroid with non-radioactive iodine to prevent internal contamination from inhaled or ingested radioactive iodine released). Despite these warnings, there were reports of small numbers of residents refusing to abandon their homes and move into evacuation centres.[348]

The Japanese authorities also identified contaminated drinking water, agricultural produce, sea water and seafood contamination as key health risks. The earthquake and tsunami caused widespread death, damage and displacement (see section 3.5.5).

Summary
For most people, the most common source of radiation over a lifetime is from natural sources (including radon and cosmic rays) and medical sources (including from x-ray, PET or CT scans). The public perception of exposure and harm from nuclear energy and nuclear warfare greatly overestimates the real levels of exposure to most people from these sources.

3.5.4. Emerging technologies

New technology can be a source of anxiety for unforeseen health effects. These concerns can be well-founded. New technologies may create a situation where, because of a lack of adequate evidence and knowledge, other cultural and social factors tend to amplify the sense of risk. Many new technologies, including nanotechnology, synthetic biology and geoengineering, fall into this category.

New technologies can be associated with specific risks of harm to health – poisoning, allergic reaction, or a chronic illness. Emerging technologies are novel and unprecedented, and there is usually a higher degree of inherent uncertainty surrounding these risks – including uncertainty in the escalation and outcome.[349] In some technologies, including synthetic biology, nanotechnology and geoengineering, small pilot experimental tests will not predict every consequence of scaling up, interactions with other drugs or organisms, or the complex interactions with ecosystems or weather systems in real world situations.

The introduction of GM food technology led to the identification of many theoretical risks to health and to the environment, including allergic reactions, gene transfer from GM food to the body or bacteria within the body, and food security threats due to the crossing of genetic material from GM crops to conventional crops. These have not been observed or realised since the widespread adoption of GM in the late 1990s in North America.

With some novel technologies, there is a risk that the harms could be irreversible and substantial. Geoengineering projects that manipulate the atmospheric composition or marine biodiversity may irreversibly alter these systems in an unpredictable way. Novel organisms designed through synthetic biology may interact with and permanently change ecosystems in ways that cannot be foreseen. This type of unknowable, potentially catastrophic risk is sometimes referred to as existential risk.

Summary
For many new technologies, such as nanotechnology, GM foods, synthetic biology and geoengineering, the potential benefits of the technologies must outweigh their risks. Where there is a high level of uncertainty associated to the risks of a technology, the precautionary principle has been adopted, for example the ban on GM foods within the EU.

Further BMA resources:
- *Genetically modified foods and health: a second interim statement.* British Medical Association (2004).[166]

3.5.5. Disasters and emergencies

A natural or man-made disaster is defined by the United Nations (UN) as: "a serious disruption of the functioning of a society, causing widespread human, material or environmental losses which exceed the ability of the affected society to cope using only its own resources." Disasters are rare but severe events that overwhelm the local infrastructure of a community, including its healthcare system.

Man-made disasters include terrorist attacks and nuclear radiation events. Natural disasters are related to a particular hazard, including an earthquake, hurricane, flood or heatwave. The event itself is the hazard, and will vary in intensity, duration, scale and magnitude. The resulting damage is the harm or injury to humans, and damage to property. The impact of a disaster is the total effect that the event has on a society; it is dependent on the preparedness and vulnerability of the society and the environment.[94]

Natural disasters are increasing in frequency, in part due to climate change (see section 3.5.6).[350] They are affecting a greater number of people, not least because more people are living in vulnerable areas, including on flood plains, hurricane-prone coastal areas, and earthquake fault lines. The economic costs of natural disasters are also increasing exponentially.[94]

Tropical cyclones

Tropical cyclones (known as hurricanes, typhoons or cyclones) are tropical storms that generate winds above 73 mph, and can be graded on a scale of intensity from 1-5. The intensity of winds is proportional to the predicted damage, and the amount of rainfall determines the severity of flooding and landslides. Flooding is the main cause of injury and death from hurricanes.

The risk of tropical cyclones varies according to geography, with coastal tropical regions most at risk, and is dependent on warm ocean temperatures, which are rising as climate change increases.[94] Due to its geography, the UK is at relatively low risk of experiencing a hurricane. Disaster preparedness for tropical cyclones can include warning and evacuation systems, and protection of property.

The cyclone that affected Bangladesh and India in 1970 caused 500,000 deaths, mainly from flooding. Hurricane Mitch resulted in 12,000 deaths in Central America from flooding and landslides in 1998.

Hurricane Katrina, which affected the Gulf Coast in the US in 2005, from Florida to Texas, was recorded as the sixth strongest Atlantic hurricane, with wind speeds of up to 125 mph. More than 1,800 people died, and property damage was estimated to be $81 billion USD. The city of New Orleans, Louisiana, and many coastal towns in Mississippi, were most affected; 80 per cent of New Orleans became flooded after flood defence systems failed.

Earthquake
Earthquakes occur as a result of energy release from the movement of the Earth's crust, creating seismic waves that cause the ground to shake. Although the Earth's geology, tectonic plates, and fault lines are well known, and it is possible to determine where earthquakes are likely to be common, it is inherently difficult to predict precisely when and where an earthquake will occur. Earthquakes cause injury and death – the most common injuries are traumatic injuries to the head and body, burns and inhalation injuries. Earthquakes cause significant destruction to local infrastructure, including hospitals, and compromise the provision of healthcare.

The magnitude of an earthquake can be measured from seismographic data and recorded on a logarithmic scale. Earthquakes of magnitude five or above can have significant impact on communities, while earthquakes of magnitude one or two may go unnoticed. The number of magnitude seven or above earthquakes per year has remained relatively stable over the past century, and is mainly determined by the thermodynamics of the Earth's core (see **Figure 36**). The impact of each earthquake is increasing, due to the increasing number of people living in vulnerable areas, and the costs of damage from earthquakes.[351]

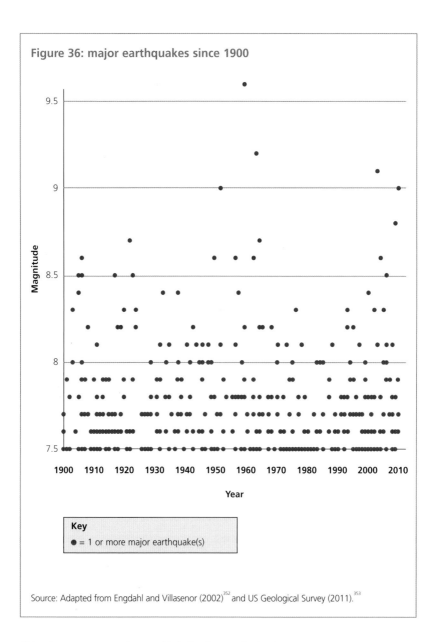

Figure 36: major earthquakes since 1900

Source: Adapted from Engdahl and Villasenor (2002)[352] and US Geological Survey (2011).[353]

The majority of earthquakes occur in the Pacific region. The UK is at relatively low risk of experiencing a high magnitude or intensity earthquake, due to its position from the mid-Atlantic ridge. The British Geological Survey estimates that the UK will experience a magnitude five earthquake once every 20 years (see **Table 6**).

Table 6: frequency of earthquakes in the UK

Magnitude	UK earthquake frequency
5	1 every 20 years
4	1 every 3-4 years
3	3 each year
2	25 each year
1	100s each year

Source: British Geological Survey (2010)[351]

Risk management for earthquakes involves ensuring the structural preparedness of buildings and infrastructure in vulnerable areas. Engineering and building design can strengthen buildings and decrease the likelihood of massive destruction from an earthquake in at risk towns and cities. Strengthening and good positioning of key services also contributes to the resilience of a community to an earthquake, by protecting utilities (gas, water, sewage, electricity), transport routes, industrial hazards, power plants and fuel storage facilities.

A number of recent significant earthquakes highlight the effect of preparedness and poverty on earthquake impact. The magnitude 7.0 earthquake that struck Haiti in January 2010 caused widespread damage: more than 230,000 people died, a further 300,000 were injured, and 1.3 million were made homeless. The earthquake damaged significant areas of the densely-populated capital Port-au-Prince and neighbouring towns and villages, destroying or damaging more than 285,000 homes. Nearly three quarters (72%) of Haiti's population live in poverty. The quality of building construction – especially in densely-populated urban areas – is very poor, and there was little or no disaster preparedness in place, which contributed to the earthquakes devastating impact.

By contrast, a magnitude 8.8 earthquake off the coast of Chile in the same year, killing approximately 570 people, did not have a comparable impact, in part due to the strict building codes in Chile, appropriate disaster preparedness and effective emergency response.

Tsunami

A Tsunami occurs from the displacement of water as a result of disturbance to the sea floor, typically from earthquake activity, underwater volcanic eruption, or landslide. The waves formed from displaced water can travel as fast as 500 mph across the ocean, and can reach a height of 10-30 metres as they reach the shore and come inland. The main damage from a tsunami is caused by its strong currents and the debris that travels with the wave.[94]

Tsunami preparedness involves implementing communication and evacuation plans, and strengthening structures that cannot be relocated. Pacific coastal regions are most at risk of tsunami, and the Pacific Tsunami Warning Centre in Hawaii aims to provide tsunami alerts for the Pacific region and globally, and to reduce the frequency of false alarms.[94] The UK is at very low risk of tsunami, and the wave heights produced by a tsunami event would be unlikely to overwhelm the UK coastal flood defence systems designed to withstand storm surges.[354]

The tsunami that affected north eastern Japan following the 9.0 magnitude earthquake off its coast in March 2011 reached more than 6 miles inland. It killed 14,000 people, with a further 11,000 missing, 130,000 homeless, and caused more than $300 billion USD of material damage. Although a warning was issued, the tsunami reached some parts of the coast within 30 minutes of the earthquake, leaving many residents unable to evacuate in time. In neighbouring areas unaffected by the tsunami, most buildings and infrastructure remained largely intact despite experiencing the high magnitude earthquake.

Flooding

Flooding is the most common type of natural disaster, accounting for more than 40 per cent of disasters and causing the greatest mortality globally per year of any natural disaster.[94] Flooding can be caused by coastal or tidal flooding, from rivers or excess rainfall.

Many areas of the UK are at high risk of flooding. Development on wetlands that normally absorb excess rainfall, or on flood plains, increases the risk of, and vulnerability to, flooding.[355] Climate change is also expected to increase the frequency and severity of flooding over the next century, including in the UK.[355] The UK Government Office for Science Foresight report *Flood and coastal defence* predicted that the number of people in the UK at high risk of flooding could increase from 1.5 million to 3.5 million, and the cost of damage could increase from £1 billion per year to £25 billion per year in the next 30-100 years.[355]

The flooding in many parts of England in the summer of 2007 affected more than 48,000 households and 7,300 businesses, led to the closure of several transport routes, and the loss of electricity, telecommunications and water supply in some areas.[95] The Environment Agency estimated that the floods cost £3.2 billion to the UK economy in damage to private and commercial property; damage to utilities, roads, and communications; flooding of agricultural land, and emergency services.[356-357]

Flood defence systems and land management are key elements of preparedness for flooding events. The Thames barrier is a major flood defence system designed to protect London and parts of southeast England against tidal surges, and flood defence systems are also located off the coast of the east of England.[355]

Extreme weather

Extreme weather, in the form of storms, extreme cold, and heatwaves, has the potential to cause harm in the UK. The storm that affected the UK on 18 January 2007 generated winds of up to 77 mph, caused widespread damage and resulted in nine deaths.[95]

Extreme cold and heavy snowfall can lead to excess winter deaths, injury and travel disruptions. Over the recent cold winters of 1999-2000 and 2008-9 in England and Wales, there were nearly 50,000 and 37,000 excess winter deaths, respectively, compared with the average for a non-winter period.[358]

A heatwave occurs in the UK where there are sustained temperatures above 32 degrees Celsius. The UK experienced a heatwave in the summer of 2003, which resulted in 2,045 excess deaths in the summer period.[359] Admissions to hospitals, sunburn, heat exhaustion and respiratory illnesses were all elevated during the heatwave. The same heatwave contributed to 14,000 excess deaths in France.[360] Older people, infants and those with chronic illnesses are at greatest risk of illness and death during heatwaves.[360]

The Met Office and the DH implement a Heat Health Watch system in the summer months as a preparedness measure to warn the public about heatwaves. Four levels of response are determined by the likelihood of a threshold daily maximum and night minimum temperatures occurring:

- level one (green) is general preparedness during the summer months
- level two (yellow) is triggered by a greater than 60 per cent chance of a threshold temperature being reached, and social and healthcare services are advised to ensure readiness to reduce harm from an upcoming heatwave.
- level three (amber) is triggered when a threshold temperature is reached for one day and consecutive night. Social and healthcare services are advised to target high risk groups to minimise vulnerability to heat waves.
- level four (red) is triggered following a prolonged or severe heatwave, where the whole population is at risk. Social and healthcare services are advised to warn the public against going out in the sun, to stay hydrated, and to keep their homes cool.

Summary
Most people, at most times, are at low risk of experiencing a natural disaster. The UK is most at risk of flooding and extreme weather events. Vivid images of disasters are readily recalled and evoke dread, leading to a heightened perception of risk.

3.5.6.   Climate change
As highlighted in the 2011 BMA Board of Science web resource *Doctors taking action on climate change*[361], climate change is a major threat to public health globally and in the UK. Rising temperatures, changing sea levels and more frequent and extreme weather patterns will lead to increased morbidity and mortality associated with changing patterns of infectious diseases, increased air pollution and UV radiation, flooding, heat waves, and food and water shortages.[339, 350, 360] Climate change will also lead to a widening of health and social inequalities

between and within countries (including the UK), with the effects most severe in developing countries and among the poorest people.[360-361] Other vulnerable groups include older people, children, subsistence farmers, traditional societies, and coastal populations.[362]

The IPCC report that climate change has already altered the distribution of certain infectious disease vectors and allergenic pollen, and increased heatwave-related deaths.[362] By the end of the 21st century, climate change is expected to:

- increase the severity and frequency of natural disasters such as heatwaves, floods, storms, fires and drought
- increase malnutrition, and affect child development
- alter the geographical range and transmission season of malaria
- increase cardio-respiratory illness and mortality from ground-level ozone.[362]

In the UK, the DH estimate that average temperatures in the UK will increase between 2.5 and three degrees before the end of the century.[360] Extreme cold weather events will decrease in frequency, but heatwaves, heavy rainfall and floods are likely to increase.[360] Higher temperatures are expected to increase ground-level ozone in the UK, leading to an increase in cardiorespiratory deaths of up to 1,500 per year, and related hospital admissions[360] The DH predict that there is a one in 40 chance of a severe heatwave in Southeast England by 2012, resulting in an estimated 3,000 excess deaths.[360] As of the autumn of 2011, Southeast England had not yet experienced a severe heatwave.

Summary
Climate change is a major threat to global public health. It is predicted to increase the risk of, and the harm from, many natural disasters and emergencies. This includes increased morbidity and mortality associated with changing patterns of infectious diseases, increased air pollution and UV radiation, flooding, heat waves, and food and water shortages. Lack of attention to this risk may result from a sense that climate change is a future rather than immediate event, and that there is little that individuals can do that would have a significant impact.[37] It would be unfortunate if we so lightly accepted the consequences for our children and grandchildren. This neglect of large risks requiring collective action is a serious problem of current risk perception.

3.5.7. Extreme threats

Extreme events can include natural disasters, as described in the previous sections, as well as man-made disasters such as industrial accidents (see section 3.5.2), terrorist attacks, explosions, train or subway derailments, aircraft crashes or hijacks, civil war and rioting.

Many of these extreme events involve collective violence (see section 3.2.12). These violent events cause significant harm to health, and lead to injury and death, often among the civilian population not directly engaged in fighting.

Extreme violent events can involve the use of conventional explosives, and chemical or biological weapons. The 2004 BMA Board of Science report *Biotechnology, weapons and humanity II* outlines the forms of biological and chemical warfare, the dual use dilemma in biotechnology research (see also section 2.4.4), and the function and limitations of the UN biological and chemical weapons conventions (BWC and CWC, respectively) that aim to restrict the use of biological and chemical warfare in conflicts.

Terrorism

Terrorism is a form of collective violence that aims to cause mass destruction to a community, thereby instilling fear in the local and wider population. Terrorist attacks are increasingly perpetrated by highly dispersed terrorist groups with no fixed geographical location. Terrorism includes specific forms such as cyber terrorism, which has the aim of exporting, modifying or deleting sensitive information, or causing national infrastructure systems to fail. It can also be in the form of bioterrorism, which is the deliberate use of microbial agents as weapons towards civilians. As highlighted in the 2004 BMA Board of Science report *Biotechnology weapons and humanity II*, certain microbial agents that pose a high threat to human health have been identified as being at increased risk of being used in bioterrorism attacks, including anthrax, smallpox, plague, botulism, ebola, tularaemia, Lassa fever and Rift Valley fever.

The threat of terrorism as a form of collective violence is not new to the UK. The principal past domestic threat was from dissident Irish republican groups and loyalist paramilitary groups in Northern Ireland. In recent years this has been replaced by other terrorist threats, such as those in July 2005, which involved four coordinated suicide attacks on the London transport network. The Maplecroft global *Terrorism Risk Index* currently rates the UK at 'medium risk' of terrorism in 2011.[i]

In contrast to natural disaster risk modelling, risk assessment models for terrorism are underdeveloped, due to the high levels of uncertainty and complexity associated with terrorism. The parameters that determine the terrorism risk to a target – a specific location, city or country, for example – include:

- the threat to a target: the likelihood of an attack by a person or organisation that has the intent and capability of causing damage
- the vulnerability of a target: the likelihood that damage occurs to a target, in terms of death, injury, property damage, etc
- the consequence of damage: the magnitude and types of damage to a target in the event of a terrorist attack.

Uncertainty in estimating risk arises from errors in assessing or predicting the threats, vulnerability and consequences of terrorist attacks.[363]

A nation's counter-terrorism strategy aims to reduce the risk of a terrorist attack on its citizens, through prevention, mitigation, and strengthening protection against attacks. In the UK, the Home Office, Security Services and Joint Terrorist Analysis Centre (JTAC) are responsible for assessing the terrorism threat level in the UK and managing the counter-terrorism strategy (CONTEST). This strategy has four strands: *pursue*, stop terrorist attacks; *prevent*, stop people becoming terrorists; *protect*, strengthen our protection against terrorist attack; and *prepare*, mitigate the impact of attacks.

---

i Maplecroft publish reports for a number of global risks, drawing from research on a wide range of social, political, environmental and economic risk indicators.

Protection can involve securing natural infrastructure, crowded areas and UK borders. Mitigation measures include emergency response preparedness and coordination. Prevention can involve acting on intelligence, and enhancing the powers of police and security services. Several recent pieces of legislation have had this aim, including the Terrorism Act 2000; the Anti-Terrorism, Crime and Security Act 2001; the Prevention of Terrorism Act 2005; the Terrorism Act 2006 and the Counter-Terrorism Act 2008. As a practical example, x-ray backscatter scans, as previously mentioned, have been in use at Heathrow airport since February 2010, as an enhanced security measure against terrorist attacks in airports and on airplanes.

In the 21st century there has been a trend in international terrorist events towards the targeting of crowded public spaces, with the intent of causing mass injury and death. Risk management options to effectively deal with these threats are faced with the need to balance national security risks against the protection of civil liberties.

Summary
Although the terrorism threat in the UK remains significant, the risk of an individual experiencing a terrorist event in the UK remains low, relative to many other risks described in this report. Extreme threats evoke fear and dread in the population, and can lead to a focus on the horrific outcome of an event, dismissing its low likelihood (probability neglect). Risk management and counter-terrorism strategies aim to prevent, mitigate and protect against terrorist attacks.

Further BMA resources:
- *Emergency planning arrangements for the NHS in the UK – a collection of responses from the Board of Science.* British Medical Association (2006).[364]

Risk: what's your perspective? A guide for healthcare professionals

CONCLUSION

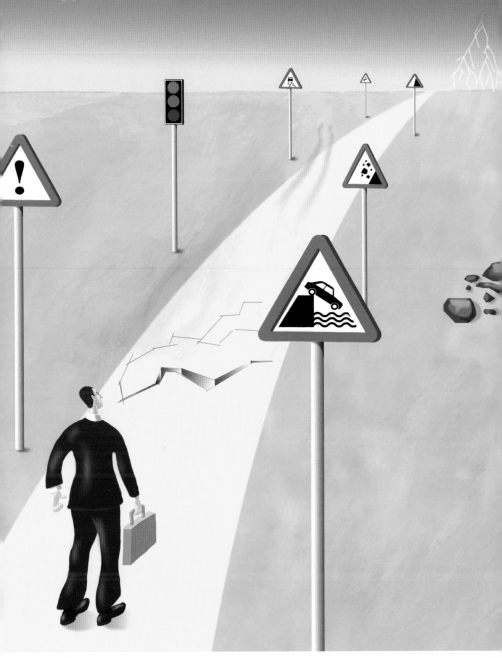

4.   CONCLUSION

This report highlights the breadth of risks that we face in everyday life, from the extremely rare to the most common. These range from smoking and alcohol use, to road traffic injuries, pandemic influenza, HCAIs, natural disasters and radiation exposure.

Nothing in life is free from risk, or completely safe. Risks can rarely be completely eliminated. Managing risks inevitably involves weighing one against another, balancing potential benefits against harm, with the aim of reducing risk to an acceptable level. Whether it is an individual seeking to manage the risks in their lives, or healthcare organisations and governments prioritising resources, a good understanding of these risks, however minor or remote, can help to put risk in perspective.

Doctors manage risk in their daily practice, whether their specialty is surgery, public health, general practice or emergency medicine. An understanding of risk – what it is, how it is measured, managed and perceived – is the foundation to understanding and putting risk into perspective.

As trusted members of society, doctors are often faced with the important role of communicating risk to patients and the public. Communicating information that is meaningful and relevant to an individual or group, in a way that is clear and simple to understand, helps people make informed choices about the risks they face. Understanding common attitudes and perceptions about risks is a key component of an effective communication strategy. This report demonstrates some effective graphical, numerical and verbal communication methods that can improve the effectiveness of risk communication. It helps doctors put the most common, and commonly feared, health risks into perspective, and support their patients in making informed, balanced decisions.

SOURCES OF FURTHER INFORMATION

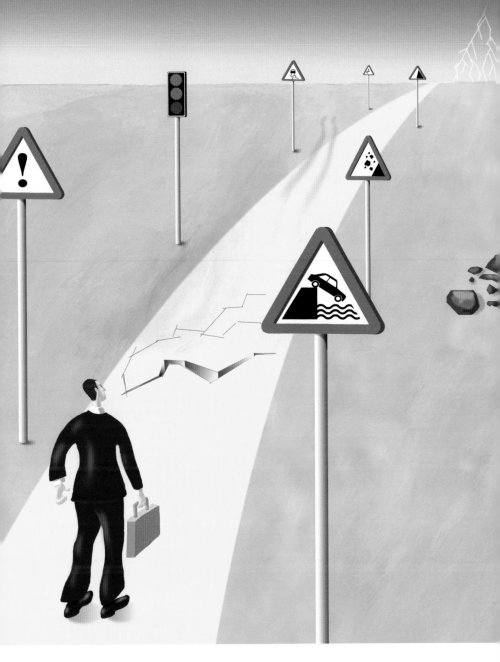

5.   SOURCES OF FURTHER INFORMATION

Bennett P, Calman K, Curtis S et al (2010) *Risk communication and public health.* Second edition. Oxford: Oxford University Press.

British Medical Association (1990) *Living with risk.* London: British Medical Association.

Cabinet Office (2010) *National risk register of civil emergencies.* London: Cabinet Office.

Ciottone GR (2006) *Disaster medicine.* Third Edition. Philadelphia: Mosby Elsevier.

Fischhoff B & Kadvany J (2011) *Risk: a very short introduction.* Oxford: Oxford University Press.

Royal Society (1992) *Risk: analysis, perception, management.* London: The Royal Society.

United States Food and Drug Administration (2011) *Communicating risks and benefits: an evidence-based user's guide.* Washington, DC: US Food and Drug Administration.

World Health Organization (2009) *The global burden of disease: 2004 update.* Geneva: World Health Organization.

REFERENCES

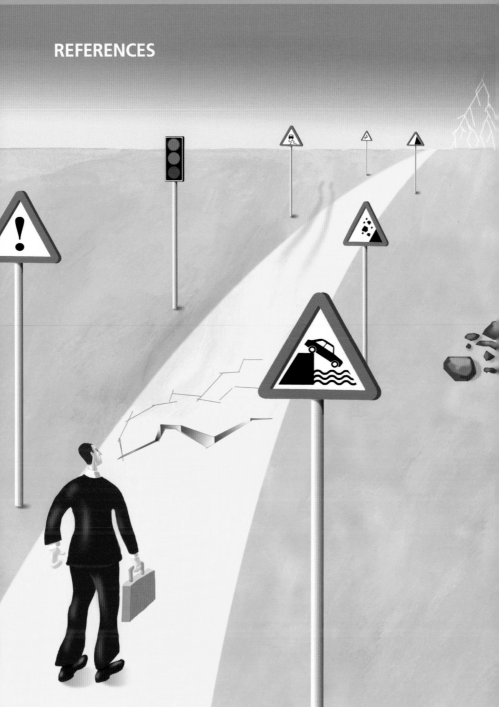

6. REFERENCES

1.   Slovic P (1987) Perception of risk. *Science* **236**: 280-5.
2.   Power M (2004) *The risk management of everything: rethinking the politics of uncertainty.* London: Demos.
3.   British Medical Association (1990) *Living with Risk.* London: British Medical Association.
4.   Bennett P, Calman K, Curtis S et al (2010) *Risk communication and public health. Second edition* Oxford: Oxford University Press.
5.   Doll R & Hill AB (1950) Smoking and carcinoma of the lung; preliminary report. *British Medical Journal* **2**: 739-48.
6.   Academy of Medical Sciences (2007) *Identifying the environmental causes of disease: how should we decide what to believe and when to take action?* London: Academy of Medical Sciences.
7.   Doll R, Peto R, Boreham J et al (2004) Mortality in relation to smoking: 50 years' observations on male British doctors. *British Medical Journal* **328**: 1519.
8.   British Medical Association (2006) *Reporting adverse drug reactions.* London: British Medical Association.
9.   Nissen SE & Wolski K (2007) Effect of rosiglitazone on the risk of myocardial infarction and death from cardiovascular causes. *New England Journal of Medicine* **356**: 2457-71.
10.   Cohen D (2010) Rosiglitazone: what went wrong? *British Medical Journal* **341**: c4848.
11.   Moynihan R (2010) Rosiglitazone, marketing, and medical science. *British Medical Journal* **340**: c1848.
12.   United States Senate Committee on Finance (2010) *Staff report on GlaxoSmithKline and the diabetes drug Avandia.* Washington DC: United States Senate Committee on Finance.
13.   European Medicines Agency press release (23.09.2010) European medicines agency recommends suspension of avandia, avandamet and avaglim.
14.   Spiegelhalter DJ (2008) Understanding uncertainty. *Annals of Family Medicine* **6**: 196-7.
15.   Bolton P (2008) *Statistical literacy guide – uncertainty and risk.* London: House of Commons Library.
16.   Department of Health (1989) *Report of the working party on bovine spongiform encephalopathy.* London: Department of Health.
17.   Ghani AC, Ferguson NM, Donnelly CA et al (2000) Predicted vCJD mortality in Great Britain. *Nature* **406**: 583-4.
18.   de Marco MF, Linehan J, Gill ON et al (2010) Large-scale immunohistochemical examination for lymphoreticular prion protein in tonsil specimens collected in Britain. *Journal of Pathology* **222**: 380-7.

19. Hilton DA, Ghani AC, Conyers L et al (2004) Prevalence of lymphoreticular prion protein accumulation in UK tissue samples. *Journal of Pathology* **203**: 733-9.

20. Alaszewski A& Horlick-Jones T (2003) How can doctors communicate information about risk more effectively? *British Medical Journal* **327**: 728-31.

21. Fischhoff B, Brewer NT & Downs J (2011) *Communicating risks and benefits: an evidence-based user's guide.* Washington DC: United States Food and Drug Administration.

22. Fischhoff B, Bostrom A & Quadrel MJ (1993) Risk perception and communication. *Annual Review of Public Health* **14**: 183-203.

23. The Royal Society (1992) *Risk: analysis, perception, management.* London: The Royal Society.

24. Alaszewski A (2005) A person-centred approach to communicating risk. *PLoS Medicine* **2**: e41.

25. Tversky A & Kahneman D (1974) Judgment under uncertainty: heuristics and biases. *Science* **185**: 1124-31.

26. Fischhoff B & Kadvany J (2011) *Risk: a very short introduction.* Oxford: Oxford University Press.

27. Kahneman D, Slovic P & Tversky A (1982) *Judgement under uncertainty: heuristics and biases.* Cambridge: Cambrigde University Press.

28. Weinstein N (1980) Unrealistic optimism about future life events. *Journal of Personality and Social Psychology* **39**: 806-20.

29. Weinstein ND (1989) Optimistic biases about personal risks. *Science* **246**: 1232-3.

30. Weinstein ND, Marcus SE & Moser RP (2005) Smokers' unrealistic optimism about their risk. *Tobacco Control* **14**: 55-9.

31. Fischhoff B, Gonzalez RA, Lerner JS et al (2005) Evolving judgments of terror risks: foresight, hindsight, and emotion. *Journal of Experimental Psychology: Applied* **11**: 124-39.

32. Johnson BB (2010) Trust and terrorism: citizen responses to anti-terrorism performance history. *Risk Analysis* **30**: 1328-40.

33. Fischhoff B (1975) Hindsight is not equal to foresight: the effect of outcome knowledge on judgment under uncertainty. *Journal of Experimental Psychology: Human Perception and Performance* **1**: 288-99.

34. Sunstein CR (2003) Terrorism and probability neglect. *Journal of Risk and Uncertainty* **26**: 121-36.

35. Sunstein CR & Zeckhauser R (2010) Dreadful possibilities, neglected probabilities In: Michel-Kerjan E, Slovic P (ed) *The irrational economist. Making decisions in a dangerous world*. New York: Public Affairs Books.

36. Slovic P, Finucane ML, Peters E et al (2004) Risk as analysis and risk as feelings: some thoughts about affect, reason, risk, and rationality. *Risk Analysis* **24**: 311-22.

37. Pidgeon N & Fischoff B (2011) The role of social and decision sciences in communicating uncertain climate risks. *Nature Climate Change* **1**: 35-41.

38. Finucane ML, Alhakami A, Slovic P et al (2000) The affect heuristic in judgments of risks and benefits. *Journal of Behavioral Decision Making* **13**: 1-17.

39. Slovic P, Peters E, Finucane ML et al (2005) Affect, risk, and decision making. *Health Psychology* **24**: s35-40.

40. Bechara A, Damasio H & Damasio AR (2000) Emotion, decision making and the orbitofrontal cortex. *Cerebral Cortex* **10**: 295-307.

41. Alhakami AS & Slovic P (1994) A psychological study of the inverse relationship between perceived risk and perceived benefit. *Risk Analysis* **14**: 1085-96.

42. British Medical Association (2007) *The use of sunbeds.* London: British Medical Association.

43. National Academy of Sciences (2010) *The science of adolescent risk taking: workshop report.* Washington, DC: National Academy of Sciences.

44. Simons-Morton B, Chen R, Abroms L et al (2004) Latent growth curve analyses of peer and parent influences on smoking progression among early adolescents. *Health Psychology* **23**: 612-21.

45. Rodham K, Brewer H, Mistral W et al (2006) Adolescents' perception of risk and challenge: a qualitative study. *Journal of Adolescence* **29**: 261-72.

46. Schneider S & Kramer H (2010) Who uses sunbeds? A systematic literature review of risk groups in developed countries. *Journal of the European Academy of* Dermatology and Venereology **24**: 639-48.

47. The Health and Social Care Information Centre (2010) *Smoking, drinking and drug use among young people in England in 2009.* Leeds: The Health and Social Care Information Centre.

48. Simons-Morton BG (2004) The protective effect of parental expectations against early adolescent smoking initiation. *Health Education Research* **19**: 561-9.

49. Imamura M, Tucker J, Hannaford P et al (2007) Factors associated with teenage pregnancy in the European Union countries: a systematic review. *European Journal of Public Health* **17**: 630-6.

50. Gigerenzer G & Edwards A (2003) Simple tools for understanding risks: from innumeracy to insight. *British Medical Journal* **327**: 741-4.

51. Tversky A & Kahneman D (1981) The framing of decisions and the psychology of choice. *Science* **211**: 453-8.

52. Brewer NT, Chapman GB, Gibbons FX et al (2007) Meta-analysis of the relationship between risk perception and health behavior: the example of vaccination. *Health Psychology* **26**: 136-45.

53. Kasperson R, Renn O & Slovic P (1988) The social amplification of risk: a conceptual framework. *Risk Analysis* **8**: 177-87.

54. Breakwell GM (2000) Risk communication: factors affecting impact. *British Medical Bulletin* **56**: 110-20.

55. Wakefield AJ, Murch SH, Anthony A et al (1998) Ileal-lymphoid-nodular hyperplasia, non-specific colitis, and pervasive developmental disorder in children. *Lancet* **351**: 637-41.

56. Gross L (2009) A broken trust: lessons from the vaccine-autism wars. *PLoS Biology* **7**: e1000114.

57. Deer B (2011) How the case against the MMR vaccine was fixed. *British Medical Journal* **342**: c5347.

58. Godlee F, Smith J & Marcovitch H (2011) Wakefield's article linking MMR vaccine and autism was fraudulent. *British Medical Journal* **342**: c7452.

59. Health Protection Agency (2010) *Measles notifications and deaths in England and Wales, 1940-2008.* London: Health Protection Agency.

60. The Health and Social Care Information Centre (2009) *NHS Immunisation Statistics England 2008-09.* Leeds: The Health and Social Care Information Centre.

61. Hesse BW & Shneiderman B (2007) eHealth research from the user's perspective. *American Journal of Preventative Medicine* **32**: S97-103.

62. Epstein RM, Alper BS & Quill TE (2004) Communicating evidence for participatory decision making. *Journal of the American Medical Association* **291**: 2359-66.

63. Paling J (2003) Strategies to help patients understand risks. *British Medical Journal* **327**: 745-8.

64. Moons WG, Mackie DM & Garcia-Marques T (2009) The impact of repetition-induced familiarity on agreement with weak and strong arguments. *Journal of Personality and Social Psychology* **96**: 32-44.

65. Fischhoff B (2011) Communicating about the risks of terrorism (or anything else). *American Psychologist* **66**: 520-31.

66. Schwartz LM, Woloshin S & Welch HG (2009) Using a drug facts box to communicate drug benefits and harms: two randomized trials. *Annals of Internal Medicine* **150**: 516-27.

67. www.fda.gov

68. Adams SM, Good MW & Defranco GM (2009) Sudden infant death syndrome. *American Family Physician* **79**: 870-4.

69. Blair PS, Sidebotham P, Berry PJ et al (2006) Major epidemiological changes in sudden infant death syndrome: a 20-year population-based study in the UK. *Lancet* **367**: 314-9.

70. Gilbert R, Salanti G, Harden M et al (2005) Infant sleeping position and the sudden infant death syndrome: systematic review of observational studies and historical review of recommendations from 1940 to 2002. *International Journal of Epidemiology* **34**: 874-87.

71. Nicholson PJ (1999) Communicating health risk. *Occupational Medicine* **49**: 253-6.

72. Ipsos MORI (2009) *Trust in doctors 2009: annual survey of public trust in professions.* London: Ipsos MORI.

73. Dibben MR & Davies HT (2004) Trustworthy doctors in confidence building systems. *Quality & Safety in Health Care* **13**: 88-9.

74. Galesic M & Garcia-Retamero R (2010) Statistical numeracy for health: a cross-cultural comparison with probabilistic national samples. *Archives of Internal Medicine* **170**: 462-8.

75. Fried TR, Tinetti ME, Towle V et al (2011) Effects of benefits and harms on older persons' willingness to take medication for primary cardiovascular prevention. *Archives of Internal Medicine* **171**: 923-8.

76. Malenka DJ, Baron JA, Johansen S et al (1993) The framing effect of relative and absolute risk. *Journal of General Internal Medicine* **8**: 543-8.

77. Gigerenzer G, Wegwarth O & Feufel M (2010) Misleading communication of risk. *British Medical Journal* **341**: c4830.

78. Larsson LG, Nystrom L, Wall S et al (1996) The Swedish randomised mammography screening trials: analysis of their effect on the breast cancer related excess mortality. *Journal of Medical Screening* **3**: 129-32.

79. Gotzsche PC & Nielsen M (2011) Screening for breast cancer with mammography. *Cochrane Database Systematic Review* **1**: CD001877.

80. Gigerenzer G, Mata J & Frank R (2009) Public knowledge of benefits of breast and prostate cancer screening in Europe. *Journal of the National Cancer Institute* **101**: 1216-20.

81. Lipkus IM (2007) Numeric, verbal, and visual formats of conveying health risks: suggested best practices and future recommendations. *Medical Decision Making* **27**: 696-713.

82. Peters E, Hart PS & Fraenkel L (2011) Informing patients: the influence of numeracy, framing, and format of side effect information on risk perceptions. *Medical Decision Making* **31**: 432-6.

83. Lipkus IM & Hollands JG (1999) The visual communication of risk. *Journal of the National Cancer Institute Monographs* **25**: 149-63.

84. Spiegelhalter D, Pearson M (2010) Understanding uncertainty: small but lethal. *Plus magazine* (online publication, Issue **55**).

85. Hogan MC, Foreman KJ, Naghavi M et al (2010) Maternal mortality for 181 countries, 1980-2008: a systematic analysis of progress towards Millennium Development Goal 5. *Lancet* **375**: 1609-23.

86. Royal College of Anaesthetists (2009) *Risks associated with your anaesthetic*. London: Royal College of Anaesthetists.

87. Spiegelhalter D, Pearson M & Short I (2011) Visualizing uncertainty about the future. *Science* **333**: 1393-400.

88. Peters E, Dieckmann N, Dixon A et al (2007) Less is more in presenting quality information to consumers. *Medical Care Research and Review* **64**: 169-90.

89. Rogers L, Siu SS, Luesley D et al (2009) Adjuvant radiotherapy and chemoradiation after surgery for cervical cancer. *Cochrane Database Systematic Reviews* **4**: CD007583.

90. Ancker JS, Senathirajah Y, Kukafka R et al (2006) Design features of graphs in health risk communication: a systematic review. *Journal of the American Medical Informatics Association* **13**: 608-18.

91. Galesic M, Garcia-Retamero R & Gigerenzer G (2009) Using icon arrays to communicate medical risks: overcoming low numeracy. *Health Psychology* **28**: 210-6.

92. Garcia-Retamero R, Galesic M & Gigerenzer G (2010) Do icon arrays help reduce denominator neglect? *Medical Decision Making* **30**: 672-84.

93. Health Protection Agency (2009) *Radon and public health: Report of the independent advisory group on ionising radiation.* London: Health Protection Agency.

94. Ciottone GR (2006) *Disaster medicine* (Third Edition). Philadelphia: Mosby Elsevier.

95. Cabinet Office (2010) *National risk register of civil emergencies.* London: Cabinet Office.

96. Pilkington P & Kinra S (2005) Effectiveness of speed cameras in preventing road traffic collisions and related casualties: systematic review. *British Medical Journal* **330**: 331-4.

97. Mindell JS, Watkins SJ & Cohen JM (2011) *Health on the Move 2.* Stockport: Transport and Health Study Group.

98. Health and Safety Executive (2001) *Reducing risks, protecting people.* London: Health and Safety Executive.

99. Martuzzi M & Tickner JA (2004) *The precautionary principle: protecting public health, the environment and the future of our children.* Copenhagen: World Health Organization.

100. Quiggin J (2007) *Complexity, climate change and the precautionary principle.* Brisbane, Queensland: Risk and sustainable management group, University of Queensland.

101. United Nations (1992) *United Nations framework convention on climate change.* New York: United Nations.

102. United Nations (1992) *Rio declaration on environment and development.* Rio di Janiero: United Nations.

103. Selgelid MJ (2009) Governance of dual-use research: an ethical dilemma. *Bulletin of the World Health Organization* **87**: 720-3.

104. National Research Council (2007) *Science and security in a post 9/11 world: a report based on regional discussions between the science and security communities.* Washington, DC: The National Academies Press.

105. Parliamentary Office of Science and Technology (2009) *The dual-use dilemma.* London: Parliamentary Office of Science and Technology.

106. Cello J, Paul AV & Wimmer E (2002) Chemical synthesis of poliovirus cDNA: generation of infectious virus in the absence of natural template. *Science* **297**: 1016-8.

107. Tumpey TM, Basler CF, Aguilar PV et al (2005) Characterization of the reconstructed 1918 Spanish influenza pandemic virus. *Science* **310**: 77-80.

108. House of Commons Science and Technology Committee (2003) *The scientific response to terrorism*. London: House of Commons.

109. Calman KC (1996) Cancer: science and society and the communication of risk. *British Medical Journal* **313**: 799-802.

110. Office for National Statistics (2010) *Mortality statistics: deaths registered in 2009*. Newport: Office for National Statistics.

111. World Health Organization (2009) *The global burden of disease: 2004 update*. Geneva: World Health Organization.

112. Ezzati M, Lopez AD, Rodgers A et al (2002) Selected major risk factors and global and regional burden of disease. *Lancet* **360**: 1347-60.

113. Yach D, Hawkes C, Gould CL et al (2004) The global burden of chronic diseases: overcoming impediments to prevention and control. *Journal of the American Medical Association* **291**: 2616-22.

114. Zimmet P, Alberti KGMM & Shaw J (2001) Global and societal implications of the diabetes epidemic. *Nature* **414**: 782-7.

115. World Health Organization (2009) *Global health risks: mortality and burden of disease attributable to selected major risks*. Geneva: World Health Organization.

116. World Health Organization (2004) *The global burden of disease: 2004 update*. Geneva: World Health Organization.

117. Department of Health (2010) *Health profile of England 2009*. London: Department of Health.

118. Sasco AJ, Secretan MB & Straif K (2004) Tobacco smoking and cancer: a brief review of recent epidemiological evidence. *Lung Cancer* **45**: s3-9.

119. Vineis P, Alavanja M, Buffler P et al (2004) Tobacco and cancer: recent epidemiological evidence. *Journal of the National Cancer Institute* **96**: 99-106.

120. Nutt D, King LA, Saulsbury W et al (2007) Development of a rational scale to assess the harm of drugs of potential misuse. *Lancet* **369**: 1047-53.

121. Office for National Statistics (2009) *Smoking-related behaviour and attitudes, 2008/9. Opinions survey report no. 40*. Newport: Office for National Statistics.

122. The Marmot Review (2010) *Fair society, healthy lives: strategic review of health inequalities in England post 2010*. London: The Marmot Review.

123. British Medical Association (2008) *Forever Cool: the influence of smoking imagery on young people*. London: British Medical Association.

124. British Medical Association (2007) *Breaking the cycle of children's exposure to tobacco smoke*. London: British Medical Association.

125. British Medical Association (2004) *Smoking and reproductive life*. London: British Medical Association.

126. British Medical Association (2008) *Alcohol misuse: tackling the UK epidemic.* London: British Medical Association.

127. Rehm J, Room R, Graham K et al (2003) The relationship of average volume of alcohol consumption and patterns of drinking to burden of disease: an overview. *Addiction* **98**: 1209-28.

128. Room R, Babor T & Rehm J (2005) Alcohol and public health. *Lancet* **365**: 519-30.

129. Sacco RL, Elkind M, Boden-Albala B et al (1999) The protective effect of moderate alcohol consumption on ischemic stroke. *Journal of the Americal Medical Association* **281**: 53-60.

130. Boffetta P & Garfinkel L (1990) Alcohol drinking and mortality among men enrolled in an American Cancer Society prospective study. *Epidemiology* **1**: 342-8.

131. The Health and Social Care Information Centre (2010) *Health survey for England – 2009: Health and lifestyles.* Leeds: The Health and Social Care Information Centre.

132. Office for National Statistics (2010) *Alcohol-related deaths in the United Kingdom 1991-2008.* Newport: Office for National Statistics.

133. Office for National Statistics (2011) *Alcohol-related deaths in the United Kingdom, 2000-2009.* Newport: Office for National Statistics.

134. Department for Transport (2011) *Reported road casualties in Great Britain: 2010 provisional estimates for accidents involving illegal alcohol levels.* London: Department for Transport.

135. Department for Transport (2011) *Reported road casualties Great Britain: 2010.* London: Department for Transport.

136. The Health and Social Care Information Centre (2010) *Statistics on alcohol: England, 2010.* Leeds: The Health and Social Care Information Centre.

137. The Health and Social Care Information Centre (2011) *Statistics on alcohol: England, 2011.* Leeds: The Health and Social Care Information Centre.

138. British Medical Association (2009) *Under the influence: the damaging effect of alcohol marketing on young people.* London: British Medical Association.

139. British Medical Association (2007) *Fetal alcohol spectrum disorders.* London: British Medical Association.

140. Nutt DJ, King LA & Phillips LD (2010) Drug harms in the UK: a multicriteria decision analysis. *Lancet* **376**: 1558-65.

141. van Amsterdam J, Opperhuizen A, Koeter M et al (2010) Ranking the harm of alcohol, tobacco and illicit drugs for the individual and the population. *European Addiction Research* **16**: 202-7.

142. Davies C English L, Stewart C etal (2010) *United Kingdom drug situation: annual report to the European Monitoring Centre for Drugs and Drug Addiction (EMCDDA) 2010.* London: Department of Health.

143.   The Health and Social Care Information Centre (2011) *Smoking, drinking and drug use among young people in England in 2010*. Leeds: The Health and Social Care Information Centre.

144.   Office for National Statistics (2011) *Deaths related to drug poisoning in England and Wales, 2010*. Newport: Office for National Statistics.

145.   Health Protection Agency (2010) *Data tables of the unlinked anonymous monitoring survey of HIV and hepatitis in injecting drug users*. London: Health Protection Agency.

146.   Health Protection Agency (2011) *STI annual data tables – STI data for the UK (Table 12)* London: Health Protection Agency.

147.   Health Protection Agency (2010) *HIV in the United Kingdom: 2010 report*. London: Health Protection Agency.

148.   British Medical Association (2006) *Sexual health clinics – examples of good practice*. London: British Medical Association.

149.   British Medical Association (2008) *Sexually transmitted infections (STI) update*. London: British Medical Association.

150.   House of Commons Health Committee (2004) *Obesity: third report of Session 2003-04*. London: The Stationery Office.

151.   Whitlock G, Lewington S, Sherliker P et al (2009) Body-mass index and cause-specific mortality in 900 000 adults: collaborative analyses of 57 prospective studies. *Lancet* **373**: 1083-96.

152.   World Cancer Research Fund & American Institute for Cancer Research (2007) *Food, nutrition, physical activity and the prevention of cancer: a global perspective*. Washington American Institute for Cancer Research.

153.   Foresight (2008) *Tackling obesities: future choices – project report*. London: Government Office for Science.

154.   British Medical Association (2005) *Preventing childhood obesity*. London: British Medical Association.

155.   British Medical Association (2009) *Early life nutrition and lifelong health*. London: British Medical Association.

156.   The Health and Social Care Information Centre (2010) *Statistics on obesity, physical activity and diet: England, 2010*. Leeds: The Health and Social Care Information Centre.

157.   Department of Health (2011) *Start active, stay active. A report on physical activity for health from the four home countries' Chief Medical Officers*. London: Department of Health.

158.   Parliamentary Office of Science and Technology (2001) *Health benefits of physical activity*. London: The Stationery Office.

159.   Department of Health (2009) *Health survey for England 2008: Physical activity and fitness*. London: Department of Health.

160.   British Medical Association (2009) *Transport and health*. London: British Medical Association.

161.   Parliamentary Office of Science and Technology (1999) *Hormones in beef.* London: Parliamentary Office of Science and Technology.

162.   European Commission Scientific Committee on Veterinary Measures Relating to Public Health (1999) *Opinion of the scientific committee on veterinary measures relating to public health: assessment of potential risks to human helath from hormone residues in bovine meat and meat products.* Brussels: European Commission.

163.   European Commission Scientific Committee on Veterinary Measures Relating to Public Health (2002) *Opinion of the scientific committee on veterinary measures relating to public health: review of previous SCVPH opinions of 30 April 1999 and 3 May 2000 on the potential risks to human health from hormone residues in bovine meat and meat products.* Brussels: European Commission.

164.   Parliamentary Office of Science and Technology (2003) *Food poisoning.* London: Parliamentary Office of Science and Technology.

165.   Health Protection Agency (2011) *Foodborne outbreaks reported to the Health Protection Agency, England and Wales, 1992-2010.* London: Health Protection Agency.

166.   British Medical Association (2004) *Genetically modified foods and health: a second interim report.* London: British Medical Association.

167.   www.un.org/millenniumgoals

168.   Royal College of Psychiatrists (2011) *Postnatal depression.* London: Royal College of Psychiatrists.

169.   Skakkebaek NE, Rajpert-De Meyts E & Main KM (2001) Testicular dysgenesis syndrome: an increasingly common developmental disorder with environmental aspects. *Human Reproduction* **16**: 972-8.

170.   Europa press release (31.05.2011) Bisphenol A: EU ban on baby bottles to enter into force tomorrow.

171.   Kelly YJ, Sacker A, Gray R et al (2010) Light drinking during pregnancy: still no increased risk for socioemotional difficulties or cognitive deficits at 5 years of age? *Journal of Epidemiology and Community Health* published online doi:10.1136/jech.2009.103002.

172.   Office for National Statistics (2010) *Childhood, infant and perinatal mortality in England and Wales, 2008.* Newport: Office for National Statistics.

173.   Office for National Statistics (2011) *Child mortality statistics, 2009.* Newport: Office for National Statistics.

174.   Office for National Statistics (2010) *Less advantaged children at most risk of accidental or violent death.* Newport: Office for National Statistics.

175.   British Medical Association (1999) *Growing up in Britain: ensuring a healthy future for our children* London: British Medical Association.

176. Conn JM, Annest JL & Gilchrist J (2003) Sports and recreation related injury episodes in the US population, 1997-99. *Injury Prevention* **9**: 117-23.

177. Dempsey RL, Layde PM, Laud PW et al (2005) Incidence of sports and recreation related injuries resulting in hospitalization in Wisconsin in 2000. *Injury Prevention* **11**: 91-6.

178. Finch C, Valuri G & Ozanne-Smith J (1998) Sport and active recreation injuries in Australia: evidence from emergency department presentations. *British Journal of Sports Medicine* **32**: 220-5.

179. British Medical Association (2008) *Boxing*. London: British Medical Association.

180. British Medical Association (2011) *Doctors providing medical care at sporting events*. London: British Medical Association.

181. British Medical Association (2001) *Injury prevention*. London: British Medical Association.

182. British Medical Association (1993) *The boxing debate*. London: British Medical Association.

183. Department for Communities and Local Government (2011) *Fire statistics monitor*. London: Department for Communities and Local Government.

184. Department for Communities and Local Government (2009) *Fire statistics: United Kingdom, 2007*. London: Department for Communities and Local Government.

185. World Health Organization (2002) *World report on violence and health*. Geneva: World Health Organization.

186. Home Office (2010) *Crime in England and Wales 2009/10: findings from the British crime survey and police recorded crime (second edition)*. London: Home Office.

187. Royal College of Psychiatrists (2010) *Child abuse and neglect: the emotional effects*. London: Royal College of Psychiatrists.

188. National Society for the Prevention of Cruelty to Children (2011) *Prevalence and incidence of child abuse and neglect: Key child protection statistics*. London: National Society for the Prevention of Cruelty to Children.

189. Radford L, Corral S, Bradley C et al (2011) *Child abuse and neglect in the UK today*. London: National Society for the Prevention of Cruelty to Children.

190. British Medical Association (2010) *Violence and health*. London: British Medical Association.

191. Ministry of Defence (2011) *United Kingdom defence statistics 2011*. London: Ministry of Defence.

192. British Medical Association (2007) *Domestic abuse*. London: British Medical Association.

193. Health and Safety Executive and National Statistics (2009) *Health and safety statistics 2008/09*. London: Health and Safety Executive.

194. Health Protection Agency (2011) *Risk of solid cancers following radiation exposure: estimates for the UK Population. RCE 19 report of the independent advisory Group on ionising radiation* London: Health Protection Agency.

195. Mehta P & Smith-Bindman R (2011) Airport full-body screening: what is the risk? *Archives of Internal Medicine* **171**: 1112-5.

196. Health and Safety Executive (2010) *The burden of occupational cancer in Great Britain.* London: Health and Safety Executive.

197. Smith A, Sarbjit J, Wadsworth E et al (2000) *The scale of occupational stress: the Bristol stress and health at work study.* London: Health and Safety Executive.

198. British Medical Association (2010) *Health effects of working unsocial hours and shift work.* London: British Medical Association.

199. Arendt J (2010) Shift work: coping with the biological clock. *Occupational Medicine* **60**: 10-20.

200. Waddell G & Burton K (2006) *Is working good for your health and well-being?* London: Department for Work and Pensions.

201. Fox AJ & Adelstein AM (1978) Occupational mortality: work or way of life? *Journal of Epidemiology and Community Health* **32**: 73-8.

202. Black C (2008) *Working for a healthier tomorrow: Dame Carol Black's review of the health of Britain's working age population.* London: Department for Work and Pensions.

203. Head J, Martikainen P, Kumari M et al (2002) *Work environment, alcohol consumption and ill-health: The Whitehall II Study.* London: Health and Safety Executive.

204. Friends of the Earth & The Marmot Review Team (2011) *The health impacts of cold homes and fuel poverty.* London: Friends of the Earth & The Marmot Review Team.

205. Parliamentary Office of Science and Technology (2010) *UK indoor air quality* London: Parliamentary Office of Science and Technology.

206. Committee on the Medical Effects of Air Pollutants (2010) *Long-term exposure to air pollution: effect on mortality.* London: Committee on the Medical Effects of Air Pollutants.

207. Department for Environment Food and Rural Affairs (2010) *Valuing the overall impacts of air pollution.* London: Department for Environment Food and Rural Affairs.

208. Glinianaia SV, Rankin J, Bell R et al (2004) Particulate air pollution and fetal health: a systematic review of the epidemiologic evidence. *Epidemiology* **15**: 36-45.

209. World health Organization (2005) *Health effects of transport related air pollution.* Copenhagen: World Health Organization.

210. British Medical Association (2003) *Housing and health: building for the future.* London: British Medical Association.

211. Cardis E, Deltour I, Vrijheid M et al (2010) Brain tumour risk in relation to mobile telephone use: results of the INTERPHONE international case-control study. *International Journal of Epidemiology* **39**: 675-94.

212. Frei P, Poulsen AH, Johansen C et al (2011) Use of mobile phones and risk of brain tumours: update of Danish cohort study. *British Medical Journal* **343**: d6387.

213. British Medical Association (2001) *Mobile phones and health: an interim report.* London: British Medical Association.

214. Health Protection Agency (2006) *Migrant health.* London: Health Protection Agency.

215. Anderson C, Story A, Brown T et al (2010) Tuberculosis in UK prisoners: a challenge for control. *Journal of Epidemiology and Community Health* **64**: 373-6.

216. World Health Organization (2007) *Health in prisons: a WHO guide to the essentials in prison health.* Copenhagen: World Health Organization.

217. Health Protection Agency Prison Infection Prevention Team (2010) *Infection inside: the prison infectious disease quarterly. December 2010 volume 6, issue 2.* London: Health Protection Agency.

218. Academy of Medical Sciences (2006) *Pandemic influenza: science to policy.* London: Academy of Medical Sciences.

219. Chowell G, Bertozzi SM, Colchero MA et al (2009) Severe respiratory disease concurrent with the circulation of H1N1 influenza. *New England Journal of Medicine* **361**: 674-9.

220. www.who.int

221. Cabinet Office & Department of Health (2008) *Pandemic flu.* London: Department of Health.

222. World Health Organization (2011) *Avian influenza factsheet.* Geneva: World Health Organization.

223. Donaldson LJ, Rutter PD, Ellis BM et al (2009) Mortality from pandemic A/H1N1 2009 influenza in England: public health surveillance study. *British Medcial Journal* **339**: b5213.

224. Hine D (2010) *The 2009 influenza pandemic.* London: Cabinet Office.

225. To KK, Wong SS, Li IW et al (2010) Concurrent comparison of epidemiology, clinical presentation and outcome between adult patients suffering from the pandemic influenza A (H1N1) 2009 virus and the seasonal influenza A virus infection. *Postgraduate Medical Journal* **86**: 515-21.

226. Cohen D (2009) Complications: tracking down the data on oseltamivir. *British Medical Journal* **339**: b5387.

227. Uyeki T (2009) Antiviral treatment for patients hospitalized with 2009 pandemic influenza A (H1N1). *New England Journal of Medicine* **361**: e110.

228. Weber JT, Nicoll A, Bridges CB et al (2010) The truth about tamiflu? Neuraminidase inhibitors in pandemic A/H1N1 flu. *British Medical Journal* **340**: c130.

229. Leung GM & Nicoll A (2010) Reflections on pandemic (H1N1) 2009 and the international response. *PLoS Medicine* **7**:e1000346.

230. Watson R (2011) MEPs criticise WHO over H1N1 pandemic advice. *British Medical Journal* **342**: d652.

231. World Health Organization (2010) *The international response to the influenza pandemic: WHO responds to the critics.* Geneva: World Health Organization.

232. British Medical Association (1997) *Road transport and health*. London: British Medical Association.

233. Department for Transport (2010) *Transport statistics Great Britain: 2009*. London: Department for Transport.

234. Department for Transport (2009) *Transport trends 2009*. London: Department for Transport.

235. Department for Transport (2011 *Reported Road Casualties Great Britain: 2010*. London: Department for Transport.

236. Jacobsen PL (2003) Safety in numbers: more walkers and bicyclists, safer walking and bicycling. *Injury Prevention* **9**: 205-9.

237. Woodcock J, Edwards P, Tonne C et al (2009) Public health benefits of strategies to reduce greenhouse-gas emissions: urban land transport. *Lancet* **374**: 1930-43.

238. de Hartog JJ, Boogaard H, Nijland H et al (2010) Do the health benefits of cycling outweigh the risks? *Environmental Health Perspectives* **118**: 1109-16.

239. British Medical Association (2009) *Driving under the influence of drugs*. London: British Medical Association.

240. British Medical Association (2010) *Promoting safe cycling*. London: British Medical Association.

241. The Health and Social Care Information Centre (2009) *Adult psychiatric morbidity in England, 2007: Results of a household survey*. Leeds: The Health and Social Care Information Centre.

242. Royal College of Psychiatrists (2007) *Physical illness and mental health*. London: Royal College of Psychiatrists.

243. Royal College of Psychiatrists (2009) *Debt and mental health*. London: Royal College of Psychiatrists.

244. Meltzer H, Bebbington P, Brugha T et al (2010) Job insecurity, socio-economic circumstances and depression. *Psychological Medicine* **40**: 1401-7.

245. Government Office for Science Foresight (2008) *Mental Capital and Wellbeing*. . London: Government Office for Science.

246. Jenkins R, Bhugra D, Bebbington P, et al. (2008) Debt, income and mental disorder in the general population. *Psychological Medicine* **38**: 1485-93.

247. British Medical Association (2011) *Psychological and social needs of patients*. London: British Medical Association.

248. British Medical Association (2006) *Child and adolescent health: a guide for healthcare professionals*. London: British Medical Association.

249. He FJ & MacGregor GA (2004) Effect of longer-term modest salt reduction on blood pressure. *Cochrane Database Systematic Reviews* **3**: CD004937.

250. Hooper L, Bartlett C, Davey SG et al (2004) Advice to reduce dietary salt for prevention of cardiovascular disease. *Cochrane Database Systematic Reviews* **1**: CD003656.

251. Jurgens G & Graudal NA (2004) Effects of low sodium diet versus high sodium diet on blood pressure, renin, aldosterone, catecholamines, cholesterols, and triglyceride. *Cochrane Database Systematic Reviews* **1**: CD004022.

252. National Centre for Social Research & Medical Research Council Human Nutrition Research (2008) *An assessment of dietary sodium levels among adults (aged 19-64) in the UK general population in 2008, based on analysis of dietary sodium in 24 hour urine samples.* London: National Centre for Social Research.

253. Ford ES & Capewell S (2011) Proportion of the decline in cardiovascular mortality disease due to prevention versus treatment: public health versus clinical care. *Annual Review of Public Health* **32**: 5-22.

254. Steptoe A, Shamaei-Tousi A, Gylfe A, et al. (2007) Socioeconomic status, pathogen burden and cardiovascular disease risk. *Heart* **93**: 1567-70.

255. Clark AM, DesMeules M, Luo W et al (2009) Socioeconomic status and cardiovascular disease: risks and implications for care. *Nature Reviews Cardiology* **6**: 712-22.

256. Cancer Research UK (2011) *CancerStats: incidence 2008 – UK.* London: Cancer Research UK.

257. Cancer Research UK (2010) *Cancer in the UK: July 2010.* London: Cancer Research UK.

258. Office for National Statistics (2001) *Cancer trends in England and Wales 1950-1999.* Newport: Office for National Statistics.

259. Antoniou A, Pharoah PD, Narod S et al (2003) Average risks of breast and ovarian cancer associated with BRCA1 or BRCA2 mutations detected in case Series unselected for family history: a combined analysis of 22 studies. *American Journal of Human Genetics* **72**: 1117-30.

260. British Medical Association (2008) *Cancer genetics.* London: British Medical Association.

261. British Medical Association (2008) *Health and ageing.* London: British Medical Association.

262. Zimmet P (2003) The burden of type 2 diabetes: are we doing enough? *Diabetes & Metabolism* **29**: 6S9-6S18.

263. Sicree R, Shaw J, Zimmet P (2010) *The global burden: diabetes and impaired glucose tolerance.* Cambridge, MA: Harvard University Press.

264. Diabetes UK (2010) *Diabetes in the UK 2010: key statistics on diabetes.* London: Diabetes UK.

265. Knowler WC, Barrett-Connor E, Fowler SE et al (2002) Reduction in the incidence of type 2 diabetes with lifestyle intervention or metformin. *New England Journal of Medicine* **346**: 393-403.

266. Tuomilehto J, Lindstrom J, Eriksson JG et al (2001) Prevention of type 2 diabetes mellitus by changes in lifestyle among subjects with impaired glucose tolerance. *New England Journal of Medicine* **344**: 1343-50.

267. Bazzano LA, Serdula M & Liu S (2005) Prevention of type 2 diabetes by diet and lifestyle modification. *Journal of the American College of Nutrition* **24**: 310-9.

268. Deshpande AD, Harris-Hayes M & Schootman M (2008) Epidemiology of diabetes and diabetes-related complications. *Physical Therapy* **88**: 1254-64.

269. British Medical Association (2004) *Diabetes mellitus: an update for healthcare professionals.* London: British Medical Association.

270. Ferri CP, Prince M, Brayne C et al (2005) Global prevalence of dementia: a Delphi consensus study. *Lancet* **366**: 2112-7.

271. Knapp M & Prince M (2007) *Dementia UK – a report to the Alzheimer's Society on the prevalence and economic cost of dementia in the UK produced by King's College London and the London School of Economics.* London: Alzheimer's Society.

272. Parliamentary Office of Science and Technology (2007) *Alzheimer's and dementia.* London: Parliamentary Office of Science and Technology.

273. Verghese J, Lipton RB, Katz MJ et al (2003) Leisure activities and the risk of dementia in the elderly. *New England Journal of Medicine* **348**: 2508-16.

274. Lautenschlager NT, Cox KL, Flicker L et al (2008) Effect of physical activity on cognitive function in older adults at risk for Alzheimer disease: a randomized trial. *Journal of the American Medical Association* **300**: 1027-37. [Erratum appears in Journal of the American Medical Association 2009;**301**:276].

275. Eisenstein M (2011) Genetics: finding risk factors. *Nature* **475**: s20-2.

276. House of Lords Science and Technology Committee (2009) *Genomic Medicine.* London: House of Lords.

277. US National Library of Medicine (2011) *Genetics home reference handbook.* Bethesda, MD: US National Institutes of Health.

278. Progress Educational Trust & Royal College of Nursing (2006) *A guide to genetics.* London: Progress Educational Trust.

279. Dodge JA, Morison S, Lewis PA et al (1997) Incidence, population, and survival of cystic fibrosis in the UK, 1968-95. *Archives of Disease in Childhood* **77**: 493-6.

280. McCormick J, Green MW, Mehta G et al (2002) Demographics of the UK cystic fibrosis population: implications for neonatal screening. *European Journal of Human Genetics* **10**: 583-90.

281. newbornbloodspot.screening.nhs.uk

282. Academy of Medical Sciences (2009) *Genome-wide association studies: understanding the genetics of common disease.* London: Academy of Medical Sciences.

283. Burton H, Levene S, Alberg C et al (2009) *Tay Sachs Disease carrier screening in the Ashkenazi Jewish population: a needs assessment and review of current services.* Cambridge: Foundation for Genomics and Population Health.

284. Fernandes Filho JA & Shapiro BE (2004) Tay-Sachs disease. *Archives of Neurology* **61**: 1466-8.

285. Kaback MM (2000) Population-based genetic screening for reproductive counseling: the Tay-Sachs disease model. *European Journal of Pediatrics* **159**: s192-5.

286. Hoppitt T, Pall H, Calvert M et al (2010) A systematic review of the incidence and prevalence of long-term neurological conditions in the UK. *Neuroepidemiology* **36**: 19-28.

287. Manolio TA (2010) Genomewide association studies and assessment of the risk of disease. *New England Journal of Medicine* **363**: 166-76.

288. Scuteri A, Najjar SS, Muller D et al (2005) ApoE4 allele and the natural history of cardiovascular risk factors. *American Journal of Physiology – Endocrinology and Metabolism* **289**: e322-e7.

289. Hu G & Agarwal P (2009) Human disease-drug network based on genomic expression profiles. *PLoS One* **4**: e6536.

290. Kraft P & Hunter D (2005) Integrating epidemiology and genetic association: the challenge of gene-environment interaction. *Philosophical Transactions of the Royal Society of Biologlical Sciences* **360**: 1609-16.

291. Rotimi CN & Jorde LB (2010) Ancestry and disease in the age of genomic medicine. *New England Journal of Medicine* **363**: 1551-8.

292. British Medical Association (2005) *Population screening and genetic testing.* London: British Medical Association.

293. British Medical Association (2007) *Over the counter medication* London: British Medical Association.

294. British Medical Association (2007) *Evidence-based prescribing.* London: British Medical Association.

295. Ernst E (2000) The role of complementary and alternative medicine. *British Medical Journal* **321**: 1133-5.

296. Ernst E (2007) Adverse effects of spinal manipulation: a systematic review. *Journal of the Royal Society of Medicine* **100**: 330-8.

297. Ernst E (2009) Chiropractic maintenance treatment, a useful preventative approach? *Preventive Medicine* **49**: 99-100.

298. Mills E, Montori VM, Wu P et al (2004) Interaction of St John's wort with conventional drugs: systematic review of clinical trials. *British Medical Journal* **329**: 27-30.

299. British Medical Association (2009) *Complementary and alternative medicine: what your patients may be using.* London: British Medical Association.

300. Cottrell S & Roberts RJ (2011) Measles outbreak in Europe. *British Medical Journal* **342**: d3724.

301. The Health and Social Care Information Centre (2011) *NHS immunisation statistics England 2010-11.* Leeds: The Health and Social Care Information Centre.

302. Department of Health & Health Protection Agency (2010) *Annual HPV vaccine coverage in England in 2009/10.* London: Department of Health.

303. Bellaby P (2003) Communication and miscommunication of risk: understanding UK parents' attitudes to combined MMR vaccination. *British Medical Journal* **327**: 725-8.

304. British Medical Association (2003) *Childhood immunisation: a guide for healthcare professionals.* London: British Medical Association.

305. Edwards A, Unigwe S, Elwyn G et al (2003) Effects of communicating individual risks in screening programmes: cochrane systematic review. *British Medical Journal* **327**: 703-9.

306. Tabar L, Vitak B, Chen HH et al (2000) The Swedish two-county trial twenty years later. Updated mortality results and new insights from long-term follow-up. *Radiologic Clinics of North America* **38**: 625-51.

307. Jorgensen KJ & Gotzsche PC (2009) Overdiagnosis in publicly organised mammography screening programmes: systematic review of incidence trends. *British Medical Journal* **339**: b2587.

308. Richards M (2011) An independent review is under way. *British Medical Journal* **343**: d6843.

309. Heath I (2009) Life and death. It is not wrong to say no. *British Medical Journal* **338**: b2529.

310. Royal College of Obstetricians and Gynaecologists (2010) *Amniocentesis and chorionic villus sampling: greet-top guideline No. 8.* London: Royal College of Obstetricians and Gynaecologists.

311. Royal College of Obstetricians and Gynaecologists (2006) *Amniocentesis: what you need to know.* London: Royal College of Obstetricians and Gynaecologists.

312. British Medical Association & Academy of Medical Royal Colleges (2010) *Joint statement on direct-to-consumer screening.* London: British Medical Association.

313. Lagasse RS (2002) Anesthesia safety: model or myth? A review of the published literature and analysis of current original data. *Anesthesiology* **97**: 1609-17.

314. Murphy GJ (2009) Does blood transfusion harm cardiac surgery patients? *BMC Medicine* **7**: 38.

315. The Health and Social Care Information Centre (2011) *Hospital episode statistics: total procedures and interventions 2010-11.* Leeds: The Health and Social Care Information Centre.

316. Murphy GJ, Reeves BC, Rogers CA et al (2007) Increased mortality, postoperative morbidity, and cost after red blood cell transfusion in patients having cardiac surgery. *Circulation* **116**: 2544-52.

317. Serious Hazards of Transfusion Steering Group & Royal College of Pathologists (2010) *Serious hazards of transfusion. Annual Report 2010.* Manchester: Serious Hazards of Transfusion.

318. UK Blood Services Prion Working Group (2010) *Joint UKBTS/NIBSC Professional Advisory Committee position statement: Creutzfeldt-Jacob disease.* London: UK Blood Transfusion Tissue Transplantation Services.

319. British Medical Association (2012) *Medical ethics today. Third edition.* London: British Medical Association (in press).

320. Parliamentary Office of Science and Technology (2005) *Infection control in healthcare settings* London: Parliamentary Office of Science and Technology.

321. British Medical Association (2009) *Tackling healthcare associated infections through effective policy action*. London: British Medical Association.

322. National Audit Office (2000) *The management and control of hospital acquired infection in acute NHS Trusts in England*. London: The Stationery Office.

323. Office for National Statistics (2011) *Deaths involving Clostridium difficile: England and Wales, 2006 to 2010*. Newport: Office for National Statistics.

324. Office for National Statistics (2011) *Deaths involving MRSA: England and Wales, 2006 to 2010*. Newport: Office for National Statistics.

325. British Medical Association (2006) *Healthcare associated infections – a guide for healthcare professionals*. London: British Medical Association.

326. World Health Organization (2011) *Antimicrobial resistance: factsheet No. 194*. Geneva: World Health Organization.

327. Health Protection Agency (2008) *Antimicrobial resistance and prescribing in England, Wales and Northern Ireland, 2008*. London: Health Protection Agency.

328. Henderson KL, Muller-Pebody B, Blackburn RM et al (2010) Reduction in erythromycin resistance in invasive pneumococci from young children in England and Wales. *Journal of Antimicrobial Chemotherapy* **65**: 369-70.

329. Committee on the Medical Aspects of Radiation in the Environment (2007) *Twelfth report. The impact of personally initiated X-ray computed tomography scanning for the health assessment of asymptomatic individuals*. London: Committee on the Medical Aspects of Radiation in the Environment.

330. Richards MA (2009) The National Awareness and Early Diagnosis Initiative in England: assembling the evidence. *British Journal of Cancer* **101**: s1-4.

331. Waller J, Robb K, Stubbings S et al (2009) Awareness of cancer symptoms and anticipated help seeking among ethnic minority groups in England. *British Journal of Cancer* **101**: s24-30.

332. Robb K, Stubbings S, Ramirez A et al (2009) Public awareness of cancer in Britain: a population-based survey of adults. *British Journal of Cancer* **101**: s18-23.

333. Men's Health Forum (2010) *Lives too short – the state of men's health*. London: Men's Health Forum.

334. Pruss-Ustun A, Vickers C, Haefliger P et al (2011) Knowns and unknowns on burden of disease due to chemicals: a systematic review. *Environmental Health* **10**: 9.

335. European Agency for Safety and Health at Work (2009) *European risk observatory report. Expert forecast on emerging chemical risks related to occupational safety and health*. Luxembourg: Office for Official Publications of the European Communities.

336. Broughton E (2005) The Bhopal disaster and its aftermath: a review. *Environmental Health* **4**: 6.

337. Spiegelhalter D (2011) Japan nuclear threat: the tsunami is the bigger tragedy. *BBC News* 19 March 2011.

338. Pidgeon NF, Henwood KL, Parkhill KA et al (2008) *Living with nuclear power in Britain: a mixed methods study.* Cardiff: School of Psychology, Cardiff University.

339. Bickerstaff K, Lorenzoni I, Pidgeon NF et al (2008) Reframing nuclear power in the UK energy debate: nuclear power, climate change mitigation and radioactive waste. *Public Understanding of Science* **17**: 145-69.

340. Darby S, Hill D, Auvinen A et al (2005) Radon in homes and risk of lung cancer: collaborative analysis of individual data from 13 European case-control studies. *British Medical Journal* **330**: 223-7.

341. Watson SJ, Jones AL, Oatway WB et al (2005) *Ionising radiation exposure of the UK population: 2005 review.* Oxford: Health Protection Agency.

342. Berrington de Gonzalez A, Mahesh M, Kim KP et al (2009) Projected cancer risks from computed tomographic scans performed in the United States in 2007. *Archives of Internal Medicine* **169**: 2071-7.

343. Baverstock K (2011) Chernobyl 25 years on. *British Medical Journal* **342**: d2443.

344. Peplow M (2011) Chernobyl's legacy. *Nature* **471**: 562-5.

345. Cardis E, Howe G, Ron E et al (2006) Cancer consequences of the Chernobyl accident: 20 years on. *Journal of Radiological Protection* **26**: 127-40.

346. Hatch M, Ron E, Bouville A et al (2005) The Chernobyl disaster: cancer following the accident at the Chernobyl nuclear power plant. *Epidemiological Reviews* **27**: 56-66.

347. Moysich KB, Menezes RJ & Michalek AM (2002) Chernobyl-related ionising radiation exposure and cancer risk: an epidemiological review. *Lancet Oncology* **3**: 269-79.

348. Hogg C (2011) Some still refuse to leave Fukushima exclusion zone. *BBC News* 28 March 2011.

349. Kuzma J, Priest S (2010) Nanotechnology, risk, and oversight: learning lessons from related emerging technologies. *Risk Analysis* **30**: 1688-98.

350. Intergovernmental Panel on Climate Change (2007) *Contribution of working groups I, II and III to the fourth assessment report of the Intergovernmental Panel on Climate Change.* Geneva: Intergovernmental Panel on Climate Change.

351. British Geological Survey (2010) *Are yesterday's earthquakes tomorrow's disasters?* London: British Geological Survey.

352. Engdahl ER & Villasenor A (2002) Global seismicity: 1900-1999 In: Lee W (ed) *International handbook of earthquake and engineering seismology.* Amsterdam: Elsevier.

353. US Geological Survey (2011) *Magnitude 7 and greater earthquakes, 2000-2011.* Reston, VA: US Geological Survey.

354. Department for Environment, Food and Rural Affairs (2005) *The threat posed by tsunami to the UK*. London: Deparment for Environment, Food and Rural Affairs.

355. Government Office for Science Foresight (2004) *Foresight project flood and coastal defence*. London: Government Office for Science.

356. Pitt M (2008) *The Pitt review: lessons learned from the 2007 floods*. London: Cabinet Office.

357. Environment Agency (2010) *The costs of the summer 2007 floods in England*. London: Environment Agency.

358. Office for National Statistics (2010) *Excess winter mortality in England and Wales, 2009-10 (provisional) 2008-09 (final)*. Newport: Office for National Statistics.

359. Johnson H, Kovats RS, McGregor G et al (2005) *The impact of the 2003 heat wave on mortality and hospital admissions in England. Health Statistics Quarterly 25*. Newport: Office for National Statistics.

360. Department of Health & Health Protection Agency (2008) *Health effects of climate change in the UK 2008: an update of the Department of Health Report 2001/2002*. London: Department of Health.

361. British Medical Association (2011) *Doctors taking action on climate change*. London: British Medical Association.

362. International Panel on Climate Change (2007) Summary for policymakers. In: *Climate change 2007: impacts, adaptation and vulnerability. Contribution of working group II to the fourth assessment report of the Intergovernmental Panel on Climate Change*. Cambridge: Cambridge University Press.

363. RAND Centre For Terrorism Risk Management Policy (2005) *Estimating terrorism risk*. Santa Monica, CA: RAND Corporation.

364. British Medical Association (2006) *Emergency planning arrangements for the NHS in the UK – a collection of responses from the Board of Science*. London: British Medical Association.

Risk: what's your perspective? A guide for healthcare professionals